FOUNDATIONS OF
AVERSION THERAPY

FOUNDATIONS OF AVERSION THERAPY

NORMAN H. HADLEY, Ph.D.

Department of Educational Psychology
Memorial University of Newfoundland
St. John's, Newfoundland
Canada

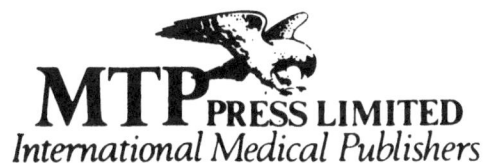

MTP PRESS LIMITED
International Medical Publishers

Published in the UK and Europe by
MTP Press Limited
Falcon House
Lancaster, England

Published in the US by
SPECTRUM PUBLICATIONS, INC.
175-20 Wexford Terrace
Jamaica, NY 11432

ISBN-13: 978-94-011-6709-3   e-ISBN-13: 978-94-011-6707-9
DOI: 10.1007/978-94-011-6707-9

Foreword

The scene is Britain in the late 40's and early 50's. More specifically, the location is the newly formed Psychology Department of the University of London Institute of Psychiatry, Maudsley Hospital. Hans J. Eysenck, then University Reader in Psychology, had an ambitious and bold plan, unheard of for those days, which he was determined to bring to fruition come what may. First, personality was to be mapped out in terms of a small number of operationally defined, measurable dimensions. Next, these dimensions would be related experimentally to their as yet to be identified underlying physiological determinants. This research was to lead to a comprehensive model of psychological, social and biological activity which would account for virtually every facet of human functioning.

To facilitate this grand scheme, Eysenck gathered around him a carefully selected team of eager young faculty and doctoral candidates among whom I had the good fortune to be included, first as a graduate student and then as a full-fledged academic. The guiding model was that of the searching student rather than the unquestioning disciple, and it was this spirit of directed but open-minded enquiry which guided us in the decades which lay ahead. That Eysenck's aspirations are not fully realized despite many years of intense endeavor does not detract from the intellectual excitement of those times and the impetus given to clinical psychology in the United Kingdom by these remarkable beginnings.

Our intellectual quest led us through the labyrinth of Pavlovian theory to the physiology of the autonomic and central nervous systems, the writings of Hull, Spence, and other learning theorists and a host of interlocking, sequentially planned laboratory studies. But this academic interest in research was soon to be tempered by reality and the exigencies of the times. As an after-

math of an exhausting war, the need for psychological services
was great and the available resources small. The rapid social
changes taking place added to the complexities of the situation,
placing further stresses upon Britain's meagre facilities. Many
problems were facing the nascent profession of clinical psychology
and, indeed, the mental health field at large.

Not only material and professional resources were lacking.
We also had little in the way of data or validated procedures to
strengthen our skimpy therapeutic armamentarium. Mental health
intervention consisted primarily of the ministrations of social workers and other caring individuals, together with a limited range
of sedative and stimulant medications. As far as formal therapy
was concerned, and this was largely in the hands of physicians,
all interventions were predicated upon untested but widely accepted psychoanalytic "truths." Clinical psychology, such as it was,
rested entirely upon these uneasy foundations and the psychological leaders in the clinical arena were virtually all psychiatrists —
Murray, Roschach, Freud, Jung and Adler, to name but a few.

Contrast this dismal state of affairs nationwide with the vital-
ity of Eysenck's visionary research program at the Maudsley. How
could this ferment and creativity be harnessed to make clinical
psychology a socially useful as well as scholarly viable discipline?
Could we develop a data-based model of clinical psychology which
stemmed out of our training as objective behavioral scientists rather
than the subjectivism of the alien tradition of psychoanalysis? If
not, as far as clinical psychology as an applied science was concerned, our years of training in the scientific study of behavior,
the generally accepted definition of psychology, would all have
been in vain.

It was the attempt to resolve this dilemma that gave rise to
what may be aptly described as the Maudsley strain of behavior
therapy, an approach which characterizes large segments of behavior therapy to this day. While contemporary behavior therapy
has numerous roots — documented in greater detail in successive
volumes of the *Annual Review of Behavior Therapy* — and this
tradition is but one among many, as far as I was concerned it was
this particular set of events which fueled the decades of clinical
and research endeavors in which I later became involved.

When the Association for Advancement of Behavior Therapy
came into being in the United States some 15 years later, it was
no accident that the name of the organization was modeled upon
the British Association for Advancement of Science. In so doing,

our declared aims were twofold: to promote an objective and scholarly advancement of knowledge and to base clinical practice upon a firm foundation of theory and research. It was hoped that the importance of being theoretical would be recognized as a primary obligation in the quest for clinical efficacy. Practical derivations were to stem out of the systematic investigation of hypotheses derived from a theoretical model, at first in the laboratory and then in the clinic. By way of compromise and the exigencies of reality, we were prepared to accept a rigorously applied empiricism as an interim strategy to "get things going" while our more painstaking rational approach was underway. This stood out in sharp contrast to the notional, anti-intellectual flavor which dominated clinical psychology in those early days – a way of thinking which is still proudly heralded as a desirable model in many parts of the psychological world!

Why am I relating this esoteric fragment of history? If all or even much of behavior therapy were now a science which lived up to these early expectations, there would be little need to make the point. Unfortunately, not all behavior therapists are true to this heritage. In certain, fortunately few, circles, intuition, hearsay and impressionism still vie with observation, theory and data as a conceptual springboard for therapeutic intervention. It is particularly refreshing, therefore, to encounter a book whose primary purpose is to take one particular facet of behavior therapy, aversion therapy, and relate it to a laboratory-based framework in which the evidence is carefully dissected and evaluated.

Aversion therapy remains a sensitive issue on numerous accounts and it behooves the behavioral clinician contemplating its use to proceed with caution. First, it is essential to be thoroughly familiar with the intricacies, strengths and weaknesses of the theory, data and research upon which the practice of aversion therapy is predicated. Second, it is important to avoid aversion techniques deployed in isolation rather than as part of a planned program involving positive as well as negative strategies. Third, an aversion or punishment procedure (the two terms are essentially synonymous) should be used only when the available evidence suggests on theoretical, research and pragmatic grounds that, for a particular purpose, it is the most acceptable alternative. Fourth, decisions with respect to usage should never be predicated upon the say-so of the therapist alone.

Despite the best of intentions, aversion therapy remains a misunderstood and misinterpreted aspect of contemporary behavior

therapy to-date and it is important that practitioners be sensitive
to the social, ethical and societal ramifications of aversion therapy
as well as the "hard" data. Positive reinforcement, negative reinforcement and punishment are three terms with precisely defined
meanings which are often at variance with those attributed to them
by the general public. Sad to relate, many psychologists are
themselves unclear about these concepts. For the behavioral
scientist, punishment is the presentation of an aversive event or
the removal of a positive event following a response which decreases the frequency of an undesired response. This definition
often conflicts with popular usage. In common parlance, punishment refers to a penalty imposed for performing a socially unac-
cepted act. It has, by and large, unhealthy connotations: a
painful mixture of personal gratification to the punisher or injured
party, retribution, coersion or "just reward" for some misdemean-
or. This is very different from punishment as used by the behavior therapist, where the primary intent is to decrease the frequency of an undesired response. (Who decides what is "undesired" is, of course, an issue which is usually glossed over.)

As far as the mundane circumstances of everyday living are
concerned, most human learning is dependent upon punishment
in some form or another: major and minor setbacks occur, paint
pots fall off ladders, provoked dogs bite and, presumably as a consequence, our subsequent behavior is altered accordingly. The
forté of the sophisticated behavior therapist lies in his or her
skillful adaptation of these principles to a comprehensive behavioral intervention program for coping with the more meaningful complexities of life which makes occasional use of these limited strategies if and as need be.

If this were all that there were to it, there would be no public
outcry against the use of aversion techniques by behavior therapists, but there is. Much has been written about this unfortunate
situation, how it came about and what to do about it. It may well
be the readily demonstrable potency of behavior therapy which
contributes, in part, to the fears of the lay public. Additionally,
terminology such as "punishment" and "aversion" do not help mat-
ters, nor do the simplistic practices and brash claims of certain
behavior therapists.

On the more positive side, most behavior therapists are hum-
anistically inclined towards both their clients and society at large.
Punishment is never used in isolation. It is always part of a carefully planned total program in which positive reinforcements are
concurrently applied. The use of therapeutic punishment is neith-

er inherently evil nor inhumane and it is inappropriate to take
an intransigent position either for or against the use of punishment. The selection of a punishment or a reinforcement program
is not an either/or decision. If used at all — and under most circumstances therapeutic punishment is contraindicated — the decision to employ a specific aversion conditioning procedure in any
particular situation rests upon many factors.

First comes the careful appraisal of available data with respect
to the clinical efficacy of a particular aversion procedure when
used as part of a comprehensive program of behavioral intervention geared to a specific patient population. Second, as a behavioral scientist, the behavior therapist must be fully cognizant of
aversion conditioning's research basis. Last, but far from least,
the practitioner has to be sensitive to the complex legal and ethical issues which permeate this troublesome area, to his or her own
personal motives in suggesting the use of punishment, and to
the various guidelines which have been promulgated at one time or
another.

Much has been written, and is being written, about the inte-
gration of aversion conditioning into a comprehensive behavior
therapy program and the ethical and legal issues involved. In
so doing, experimental foundations, theoretical models and research data tend to be overlooked. It may be that behavior therapists have strayed too far from their foundations and forgotten
their origins. In this respect, Norman Hadley's book offers a
needed corrective. A careful reading of these pages sheds light
upon the neglected principles of classical and instrumental conditioning and their application in clinical research. Even more
to the point, these developments are related to specific theoretical
interpretations which are of direct relevance to contemporary behavior therapy. Finally, attention is drawn to certain theories
of conditioning and personality and their implications for behavior
therapy. Interestingly, Eysenck's neglected formulations with
respect to the complex relationships between personality — an un-
popular popular concept in behavioral circles if ever there was
one —, conditioning and therapy feature prominently in this over-
view and so we have come full circle. I feel as if I am back in
those early days at the Maudsley — but with the added benefits
of the knowledge that we now have and the many developments
which have occurred.

This monograph is a succinct and critical documentation of
the complex relationships between learning theory and personality

as applied to aversion conditioning. It also revives a neglected
tradition which demands our serious attention.

Cyril M. Franks
Distinguished Professor
Graduate School of Applied and
Professional Psychology
Rutgers University

Preface

   This book is written for students of graduate and advanced
undergraduate courses in behavior therapy and for the applied
researcher or clinician in aversion behavior therapy. The intent
is not to review the entire field of aversive conditioning and aversion therapy but to (a) identify and outline theoretical issues,
principles, and procedures of Pavlovian and instrumental learning
paradigms, (b) examine the learning theory and research related
to aversion therapy, including escape and avoidance learning,
(c) describe and critique the screening and masking procedures
for treating self-injurious and self-stimulatory behaviors, (d)
discuss a number of specific theoretical interpretations to account
for the effectiveness of aversion therapy, and (e) study the relationship between personality and conditionability.
   A thorough understanding of the theoretical bases of aversion
therapy and knowledge of research studies is essential for the
clinician to not only deliver effective therapy but to anticipate
and avoid ethical problems and potentially harmful effects. The
characteristics, advantages, and limitations of various aversive
stimuli are studied because an awareness of these factors is important in selecting an effective stimulus for use in aversion therapy.
In addition, potential problems of using a relief stimulus in aversion therapy are examined. In the chapter on personality and
conditionability, emphasis is on Eysenck's theory of personality.
It is anticipated that this discussion will alert the therapist to the
influence of personality variables such as extraversion, introversion, and neuroticism on conditionability.
   My book on aversion therapy would be incomplete without including several additional topics specific to faradic aversion therapy such as safe and unsafe points for attaching electrodes, pain
thresholds, the use of a portable shocker for self-administered
treatment, and guidelines for constructing a faradic stimulus
shocker.

Norman H. Hadley

Acknowledgments

I am deeply indebted to Mrs. Millicent Bradbury, Mrs. Barbara Eddy, Ms. Eloise Sainsbury, Mrs. Barbara Kelland, and Ms. Joan Ritcey of the Queen Elizabeth II Library at Memorial University of Newfoundland for painstakingly assisting me in obtaining numerous materials through interlibrary loan. The assistance of the various technical services departments at Memorial University of Newfoundland is appreciated. Mr. B. Hansen, Mr. W. Wheeler, and Mr. W. Boone of Photography and Mr. S. Moss of Graphics met almost impossible deadlines in completing various pieces of work for me. I extend my sincere thanks to Mrs. Betty Morgan of the Department of Educational Psychology and the staff of the General Office, Education Building, for typing the revisions to several chapters.

I wish to thank Professor H. G. Jones of the Department of Psychology, University of Leeds, Leeds, England, for his encouragement and helpful suggestions during the preparation of the manuscript. I am especially grateful to Professor Cyril M. Franks of the Graduate School of Applied and Professional Psychology at Rutgers University for writing the foreword. A special word of appreciation is extended to Dr. Gary Jeffery, a colleague of mine at Memorial University of Newfoundland, for suggesting the title for the book. I have saved my final and most grateful thank-you for my wife Paula. Her encouragement has been undaunting and her many long hours of assistance invaluable.

The following is a list of the figures, tables, and quotations for which I have received permission to include in my book. I am indebted to the authors and publishers for allowing me to reprint excerpts from their copyrighted materials.

The quotation on pages xviii-xix is from *Behavior Therapy: Application and Outcome* by K. D. O'Leary and G. T. Wilson, Englewood Cliffs, N.J.: Prentice-Hall, 1975. Copyright© by Prentice-Hall, Inc., and reprinted with permission.

The quotation on page 8 is from *Experimental Psychology: Theory and Practice* by P. J. Dunham, New York: Harper and Row, 1977. Copyright© by P. J. Dunham, and reprinted with permission.

Figure 15, page 11, Figures 16 and 17, page 12, Figure 18, page 13, two quotations on page 14, the quotation on pages 96-97, and the quotation on page 103 are from *Psychology of Learning and Behavior* by B. Schwartz, New York: W. W. Norton, 1978. Copyright © by W. W. Norton and Company, Inc., and reprinted with permission.

The quotations on pages 15-17 are from "Pavlovian Second-order Conditioning: Some Implications for Instrumental Behavior" by R. A. Rescorla, in H. Davis and H. M. B. Hurwitz (Eds.), *Operant-Pavlovian Interactions*, Hillsdale, N.J.: Lawrence Erlbaum, 1977. Copyright© by Lawrence Erlbaum Associates, Inc., and reprinted with permission.

Figure 19 on page 18 is from *The Mechanisms of Conditioned Behavior* by W. Wyrwicka, Springfield, Il.: Charles C. Thomas, 1972. Copyright© by Charles C. Thomas, and reprinted with permission.

The quotation on page 21 is from "On the Role of the Reinforcer in Associative Learning" by R. G. Weisman, in H. Davis and H. M. B. Hurwitz (Eds.), *Operant-Pavlovian Interactions*, Hillsdale, N.J.: Lawrence Erlbaum, 1977. Copyright© by Lawrence Erlbaum Associates, Inc., and reprinted with permission.

The quotation on pages 21-22 is from "A Note on the Operant Conditioning of Autonomic Responses" by A. H. Black, B. Osborne, W. C. Ristow, in H. Davis and H. M. B. Hurwitz (Eds.), *Operant-Pavlovian Interactions*, Hillsdale, N.J.: Lawrence Erlbaum, 1977. Copyright© by Lawrence Erlbaum Associates, Inc., and reprinted with permission.

The quotations on pages 30-31 are from "Aversive Control of Behavior" by S. H. Lovibond, *Behavior Therapy*, 1970, *1*, 80-91. Copyright© by the Association for Advancement of Behavior Therapy, and reprinted with permission.

The quotations on pages 32 and 55 are from *Behavior Therapy: Techniques and Empirical Findings* by D. C. Rimm and J. C. Masters, New York: Academic Press, 1974. Copyright© by Academic Press, and reprinted with permission.

The quotation on pages 32-33 is from *Learning Foundations of Behavior Therapy* by F. H. Kanfer and J. S. Phillips, New York: Wiley, 1970. Copyright© by John Wiley and Sons, Inc., and reprinted with permission.

The quotation on pages 35-36 is from *Behavior Modification* by W. L. Mikulas, New York: Harper and Row, 1978. Copyright© by W. L. Mikulas, and reprinted with permission.

Figure 25 on page 38, Figure 26 on page 40, and the quotation on pages 40-41 are from "Response Characteristics and Control During Lever-press Escape" by H. Davis, in H. Davis and H. M. B. Hurwitz (Eds.), *Operant-Pavlovian Interactions*, Hillsdale, N.J.: Lawrence Erlbaum, 1977. Copyright© by Lawrence Erlbaum Associates, Inc., and reprinted with permission.

The quotation on page 52 and Figure 27 on page 61 are from "Electric Shock — Safety Factors When Used for the Aversive Conditioning of Humans" by W. H. Butterfield, *Behavior Therapy*, 1975, *6*, 98-110. Copyright© by the Association for Advancement of Behavior Therapy, and reprinted with permission.

The quotation on pages 53-54 is from *Psychotherapy by Reciprocal Inhibition* by J. Wolpe, Stanford, Ca.: Stanford University Press, 1958. Copyright © by Stanford University Press, and reprinted with permission.

The quotation on page 84 is from "Sexual Deviants Two Years After Electrical Aversion" by I. Marks, M. Gelder, and J. Bancroft, *British Journal of Psychiatry*, 1970, *117*, 173-185. Copyright© by The Royal College of Psychiatrists, and reprinted with permission.

The quotation on pages 86-87 is from "Aversive Conditioning: Learning or Dissonance Reduction?" by A. S. Carlin and H. E. Armstrong, Jr., *Journal of Consulting and Clinical Psychology*, 1968, *32*, 674-678. Copyright © by the American Psychological Association, and reprinted with permission.

The quotations on page 89 are from "A Theory of the Incubation of Anxiety/Fear Responses" by H. J. Eysenck, *Behavior Research and Therapy*, 1968, *6*, 309-321. Copyright © by Pergamon Press, and reprinted with permission.

The quotation on pages 89-90 and the quotation on pages 91-92 are from "The Conditioning Model of Neurosis" by H. J. Eysenck, *The Behavioral and Brain Sciences*, 1979, *2*, 155-199. Copyright© by Cambridge University Press, and reprinted with permission.

The quotation on page 91 is from "Eysenck's Theory of Incubation: A Critical Analysis" by P. J. Bersh, *Behaviour Research and Therapy*, 1980, *18*, 11-17. Copyright© by Pergamon Press, and reprinted with permission.

The quotation on pages 92-93 is from "A Theory of the Incubation of Anxiety/Fear Responses: An Alternative" by L. F. Quattlebaum, *Psychological Reports*, 1970, *26*, 747-749. Copyright © by Psychological Reports, and reprinted with permission.

The quotation on page 94 is from "Current Status of Aversion Therapy" by R. S. Hallam and S. Rachman, in M. Hersen, R. M. Eisler, and P. M. Miller (Eds.), *Progress in Behavior Modification* (Vol. 2), New York: Academic Press, 1976. Copyright© by Academic Press, and reprinted with permission.

The quotation on page 95 and Figure 28 on page 96 are from *Learning and Memory: An Introduction* by J. A. Adams, Homewood, Il.: Dorsey Press, 1976. Copyright© by Dorsey Press, and reprinted with permission.

Figure 30 on page 109 and the quotation on page 115 are from *Crime and Personality* by H. J. Eysenck, London: Paladin, 1970. Copyright© by Routledge and Kegan Paul Limited, and reprinted with permission.

Table 3, page 111, Table 4, page 120, Figure 31, page 113, and Figure 34, page 122, are from *Beneath the Mask: An Introduction to Theories of Personality* by C. F. Monte, New York: Praeger, 1977. Copyright© by C. F. Monte, and reprinted with permission.

The quotation on page 115 is from "Cortical Inhibition, Figural Aftereffect and Theory of Personality" by H. J. Eysenck, in H. J. Eysenck (Ed.), *Eysenck on Extraversion*, London: Crosby Lockwood Staples, 1973. Copyright© by Granada Publishing Limited, and reprinted with permission.

Figure 32 on page 118 and the quotation on pages 120-121 are from *The Biological Basis of Personality* by H. J. Eysenck, Springfield, Il.: Charles C. Thomas, 1967. Copyright © by Charles C. Thomas, and reprinted with permission.

Figure 33 on page 119 is from "The Influence of Stimulant and Depressant Drugs on the Central Nervous System" by R. N. Gooch, in H. J. Eysenck (Ed.), *Experiments With Drugs: Studies in the Relation Between Personality, Learning Theory and Drug Action*, New York: Macmillan, 1963. Copyright© by Pergamon Press, and reprinted with permission.

Introduction

In this volume, two intricately related facets of aversion therapy — the experimental and the clinical — are discussed. The purpose of discussing aversion therapy within a laboratory-based framework is to provide a basis from which extrapolations can be made to human behavior. Seligman (1975) asserted that "for seventy-five years experimental psychologists. . .claimed that an understanding of simple processes, lower species, and highly controlled experimental situations would shed light on real problems, in particular, human psychopathology" (p. xi). Laboratory research is beginning to yield useful information for extrapolation to human problems. As an example, Seligman (1975) forcefully argued that the learned helplessness model, which has been researched primarily in the laboratory, is as applicable to man as it is to animals. Schwartz (1978) also stressed that animal-based behavior principles are used in studying and treating human behavioral problems:

> Principles of behavior theory, derived from laboratory research with animal subjects, are being used to treat problems as diverse as alcoholism, cigarette smoking, obesity, stuttering, phobias, and learning disabilities (p. 10).

Although Schwartz's text deals mainly with the principles of learning, the author nonetheless was very aware of the importance of the extrapolation issue.

Kanfer and Phillips (1970) acknowledged that learning principles have been applied to practical human problems. The intent of their behavior therapy text was to show "how basic scientific findings from general psychology have been put to work for the betterment of human life through ingenious extrapolation" (pp. 1-2). Further support for applying findings from animal behavioral research to the study of human behavior is inherent in a statement by Staats and Staats:

In extending the [learning] principles of complex human behavior, areas of application are sometimes reached that have
not yet been sufficiently subjected .to experimentation. Never-
theless, there appears to be enough support of the basic
principles as well as a sufficient number of demonstrations
for the relevance of their extrapolations to consider a learning conception of complex human behavior to be a powerful
approach. (Staats and Staats, 1963, p. v.)

In a companion volume, called *Human Learning: Studies Extending Conditioning Principles to Complex Behavior*, Staats
(1964) reiterated his position:

A number of studies have been emerging that demonstrate
the shift from the use of human subjects for the study of
learning principles per se to the use of basic learning
principles and methods in the study of human behavior
(p. vii).

Writers of recent behavior therapy texts have also stressed
the importance of considering a learning foundation. Rimm and
Masters (1974) wrote that "there is a clear insistence that techniques designated as behavior therapy be derived from empirical
research" (p. ix).

O'Leary and Wilson (1975) provided a cautionary note on the
problems that may be associated with extrapolating from the animal literature. Referring to the work of Feldman and MacCulloch,
they emphasized that:

Feldman and MacCulloch's (1971) attempt to apply principles
from the animal conditioning laboratory, while laudable, illustrates some of the problems involved in such extrapolation.
The development of the AA [anticipatory avoidance] technique was predicated on the assumption that avoidance learning is singularly resistant to extinction (e.g., Solomon, Kamin, and Wynne, 1953), and hence least likely to result in
clinical relapse. An intermittent, random schedule was used
to prevent generalization decrement after the homosexual
avoidance habit had been acquired and so minimize extinction
of therapeutic gains (Kimble, 1961). The difficulty resides
in the fact that both avoidance conditioning and intermittent
schedules appear to derive their high resistance to extinction
from the inability of the animal to discriminate between reinforcement contingencies operating during acquisition and extinction (Wilson and Davison, 1971). Unlike the rat in the

shuttlebox, however, Feldman and MacCulloch's patients were undoubtedly aware that they could not be shocked for homosexual behavior in the natural environment; an explanation of the generalization of treatment effects must accordingly be sought elsewhere (p. 315).

While there are dangers in extrapolating, still others have expressed favorable opinions and provided evidence for the utility of this practice. Walters and Grusec (1977), for example, in their text *Punishment* have indicated that:

Much of the literature about this subject [behavior therapy] demonstrates that techniques that suppress responding in the animal laboratory also suppress responding in human beings (p. xi).

Their concluding comment reads interestingly:

But there are relatively few behavior-therapy studies that have actually extended our knowledge about the punishment process itself (p. xi).

Schwartz (1978), like Walters and Grusec, claimed that:

While attempts to apply behavior theory are not always successful, when they are, they inspire in many the confidence that more success only awaits the further development of principles of behavior theory in the laboratory (p. 10).

In this book, findings from infrahuman studies are integrated with discussions of human research to provide detailed information about several facets of aversive conditioning and aversion therapy, such as habituation, predictableness of shock, and the preparedness phenomenon. An empirical and theoretical analysis of animal lever-press escape behavior is presented because escaping the aversive stimulus in therapy often involves pressing a lever or a button. Many characteristics of animal escape and avoidance behavior are evident in aversion therapy with humans, and hence an examination of the parameters of aversive conditioning in the laboratory serves to enhance a discussion of the facets of aversion therapy.

Contents

1
Classical and Instrumental Conditioning: Principles and Procedures

The essential features of classical and instrumental conditioning will be presented to illustrate the similarities and differences between these two modes of learning.

CLASSICAL CONDITIONING PARADIGM

According to Hilgard and Marquis (1940), three features are essential to classical conditioning:

1. An unconditioned stimulus that evokes an unconditioned response.
2. A to-be-conditioned stimulus that does not initially evoke the unconditioned response.
3. Paired presentations of the conditioned and unconditioned stimuli.

In classical conditioning training trials, an identifiable unconditioned stimulus (UCS) that naturally evokes a measurable unconditioned response (UCR) is associated with a neutral stimulus. The sequence of events may be depicted as follows:

Neutral stimulus—UCS—UCR

After each block of training trials, a number of test trials are given to ascertain if an association has been learned between the neutral stimulus and the UCS. On these trials, only the stimulus to-be-conditioned is presented. If learning has occurred, the organism's response to this stimulus (CS) will be similar to the UCR that was evoked by the UCS and is technically called the con-

1

ditioned response (CR). In summary, the complete classical conditioning procedure may be conceptualized as follows:

$$CS = = = = = = = = UCS = = = = = = = = UCR$$
$$= = = = = = = = = = = = = = = = = = - CR$$

INSTRUMENTAL CONDITIONING PARADIGM

The instrumental learning paradigm may be schematized as follows (Reese and Lipsitt, 1970, p. 97):

$$S \text{------} R_o \text{------} S_1 \text{------} R_1$$

S represents an environmental stimulus, R_o the operant response, and S_1 the response-contingent stimulus. The response R_1 to S_1 is a consummatory response and the occurrence of the $S_1 \text{------} R_1$ sequence is reinforcing. Learning, therefore, in instrumental conditioning is dependent on the contingency between R_o and $S_1 \text{------} R_1$, and results in an increased probability of the rate of emission of R_o. The stimulus (S_1) in instrumental conditioning is termed a reinforcer, the function of which is to alter the strength of a response. A reinforcer may be either positive or negative. If S_1 is a positive reinforcer, it will increase the frequency of the response; if negative, it may either decrease the frequency of the operant or increase the frequency of escape or avoidance responses that terminate or prevent the presentation of an aversive stimulus. When S_1 represents the withdrawal of a positive stimulus, the conditioned response will be weakened and its frequency will gradually decline (Reese and Lipsitt, 1970; Williams, 1973).

CONDITIONING PARADIGMS: COMPARISONS AND DISTINGUISHING FEATURES

In classical conditioning, the CR is similar to the UCR; for example, conditioned salivation is very similar to the salivary response elicited by the UCS (Adams, 1976). Classical conditioning, therefore, essentially involves substituting one stimulus for another — the response elicited by the UCS comes to be elicited by the CS. In instrumental conditioning, however, the learned response is often very different from the response that is associated with reinforcement. For example, a learned lever-press response markedly contrasts with the eating of a food reward.

Autonomic behavior has traditionally been regarded as an index of classical conditioning. In the mid-1960s, however, several researchers showed that autonomic responses can be operantly conditioned. For example, in an experiment by Kimmel and Kimmel (1963), galvanic skin responses were conditioned by operant procedures. Shearn (1962) demonstrated that operant procedures can be used to condition heart rate, and salivation was operantly conditioned by Miller and Carmona (1967). In order to control for voluntary movements that may alter autonomic responses such as heart rate, other researchers (Trowill, 1967; Miller and Dicara, 1967) immobilized animals by administering the drug curare to them. Electrical brain stimulation was used as a reinforcer. Since various autonomic responses have been operantly conditioned, it appears that one of the traditional guidelines for distinguishing between operant and classical conditioning is no longer valid.

The effectiveness of intermittent reinforcement schedules in maintaining instrumental behavior is well documented in learning texts. Less attention has been given to studying the effect of partial reinforcement on classically conditioned responses. Several investigators, however, have employed partial reinforcement in their classical conditioning procedures by omitting the UCS on an arbitrary number of training trials. An example is a study by Grant and Schipper (1952) in which the human eye-blink response was classically conditioned under five different reinforcement conditions. The response extinguished most rapidly in the 0%, 25%, and 100% reinforcement groups and least rapidly in the 50% and 75% reinforcement groups. To explain these and similar findings by other researchers, Mowrer and Jones (cited in Hall, 1976) proposed that:

> Resistance to extinction is a function of the difficulty of discriminating extinction trials from acquisition trials. Thus, when the acquisition and extinction trials bear some similarity to one another, as in partial reinforcement, the subject has difficulty in determining when acquisition trials end and extinction trials begin, so that acquisition behavior continues. On the other hand, if the subject is provided with continuous reinforcement, the change to extinction trials in which reinforcement never takes place is quite marked. The result is that these trials are easily distinguished from acquisition trials, so that there is cessation of responding (pp. 133-134).

According to Williams (1973), the only way of differentiating between classical and instrumental conditioning is on the basis of experimental paradigms or procedures. The main procedural difference, from Williams' point of view, is that "in classical conditioning the reinforcement is independent of the subject's behavior whereas in operant conditioning the reinforcement is always contingent upon the subject's response" (p. 27). In addition to the procedural differences between classical and instrumental conditioning, there exist several variations *within* each conditioning paradigm. Several classical conditioning procedures will be described, while the instrumental procedures of escape and avoidance training will be discussed in another section of this monograph.

EXPERIMENTAL PROCEDURES IN CLASSICAL CONDITIONING

Varying the time interval between the CS and UCS and the order of presentation of the two stimuli are the key variables to be considered in designing classical conditioning procedures. Reference is often made in the psychological literature to simultaneous conditioning, delay conditioning, trace conditioning, backward conditioning, and temporal conditioning (Ellis, 1978; Hall, 1976; Reese and Lipsitt, 1970).

In simultaneous conditioning, the onset and offset of the CS coincides with the onset and offset of the UCS, as illustrated in Figure 1. Because of this simultaneity, the CS cannot predict the onset of the UCS. Simultaneous conditioning, according to Ellis (1978), produces little learning. An alternative to the basic simultaneous conditioning procedure is to " 'embed' the CS by timing its onset after the onset of the UCS and its offset prior to the offset of the UCS" (Dunham, 1977, p. 79), as illustrated in Figure 2.

Delay conditioning is characterized by "a delay between the onset of the CS and the onset of the UCS" (Ellis, 1978, p. 14). In one type of delay conditioning, the CS and UCS are terminated simultaneously. The essential features of this type of conditioning are depicted in Figure 3.

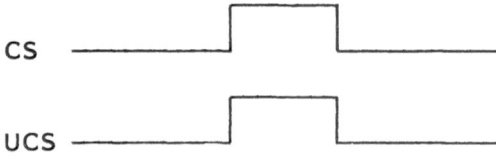

Figure 1. Simultaneous classical conditioning.

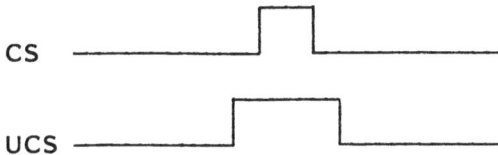

Figure 2.   Classical conditioning with CS embedded in UCS.

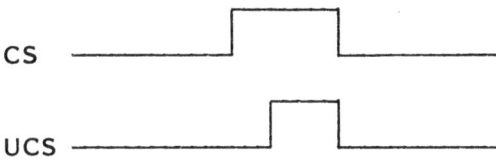

Figure 3.   Delay conditioning with simultaneous offset of the CS and UCS.

Figure 4 illustrates a second type of delay conditioning in which UCS onset coincides temporally with the offset of the CS.

Whereas the CS and UCS overlap in both simultaneous and delay conditioning, this does not occur in trace conditioning. Rather, the onset and termination of the CS occur before the onset of the UCS. The procedure is called trace conditioning "because any conditioning which occurs depends upon some trace of the CS in the nervous system since the CS is not actually present" (Ellis, 1978, p. 14). Hence the neural trace may function as the CS. This procedure is schematized in Figure 5. Ellison (cited in Hall, 1976, p. 24) found no difference between the delay and trace procedures in conditioning a salivary response in dogs when the interstimulus interval was 8 seconds. When the interval was 16

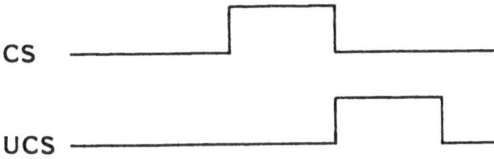

Figure 4.   Delay conditioning: UCS onset coincides with CS offset.

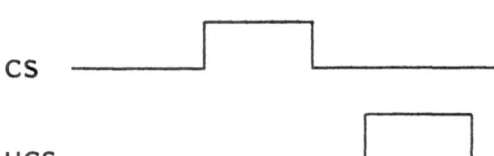

Figure 5.   Trace conditioning.

seconds, however, delay conditioning was more effective than
trace conditioning. Manning, Schneiderman, and Lordahl (1969)
found that delay conditioning was superior to trace conditioning
when ISIs of 7, 14, and 21 seconds were used. The difference in
efficacy between the two conditioning procedures, therefore, appears to be negligible for short interstimulus intervals (hypothetical example in Figure 6) but when long ISIs are employed
(Figure 7), the delay procedure is more effective (Hall, 1976).
      The UCS is always presented and terminated before the onset
of the CS in backward conditioning (see Figure 8). Because backward conditioning is difficult to obtain, it is often used as a Pavlovian control procedure (Reese and Lipsitt, 1970).
      A procedure in which a time interval functions as the CS is
called temporal conditioning. During conditioning trials, the UCS
is presented at regular intervals, for example, every 40 seconds.
Learning would be evident if the CR is emitted at fixed points
in time corresponding to the UCS presentations during training
trials. Figure 9 illustrates the procedural features of temporal
conditioning.

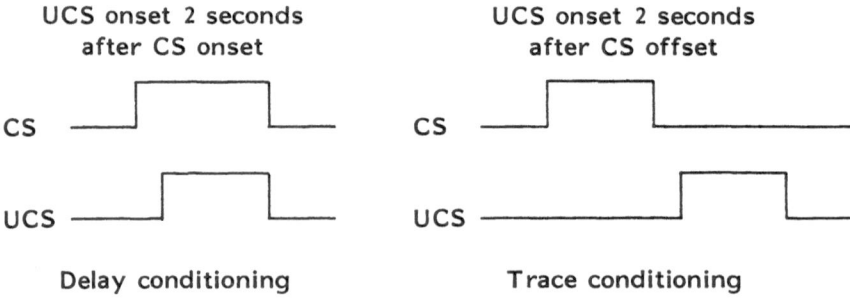

UCS onset 2 seconds   UCS onset 2 seconds
    after CS onset   after CS offset

Delay conditioning   Trace conditioning

Figure 6.   Short ISI: Negligible difference between delay and trace
conditioning in producing a CR.

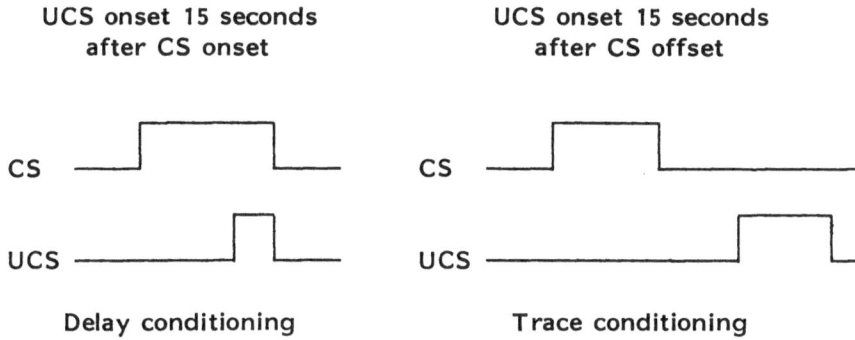

UCS onset 15 seconds   UCS onset 15 seconds
   after CS onset   after CS offset

CS   CS

UCS   UCS

Delay conditioning   Trace conditioning

Figure 7. Long ISI: Delay conditioning more effective than trace conditioning in producing a CR.

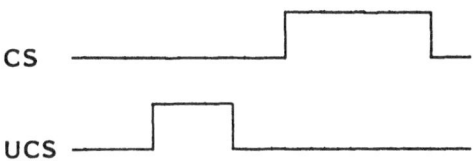

CS

UCS

Figure 8. Backward conditioning.

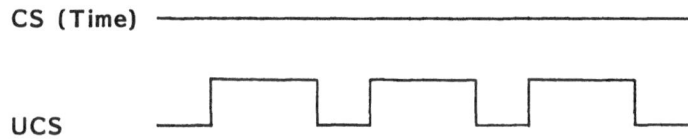

CS (Time)

UCS

Figure 9. Temporal conditioning.

CONTROL PROCEDURES IN CLASSICAL CONDITIONING

One critical experimental question with regard to classical conditioning procedures is "What behavior changes do or do not result from the temporal pairing of the CS and UCS?" It is possible that the CR may be learned because of factors other than the CS-UCS pairing. Dunham (1977) has cogently distinguished between two contaminating influences:

Pseudoconditioning. . .is a term psychologists use to imply
that a "true" association has not been learned. Specifically,
pseudoconditioning refers to cases where a stimulus other than
the UCS will elicit the UCR, even though that stimulus has
never been directly paired with the UCS.

A similar problem can occur when you use a CS that, by
itself, will elicit responses similar to the UCR to be measured
during conditioning. Although it is not likely, a tone CS
might elicit a small amount of salivation when heard by the
subject. If subsequent exposure to CS-UCS pairings simply
augments the subject's normal tendency to salivate in response
to the tone CS, there is reason to suspect that we might not
be observing the formation of a new connection. This phenomenon, called *sensitization*, is assumed to augment naturally
occurring responses to the CS and is often very difficult to
detect (p. 73).

In order to determine the effects that are directly produced
by the CS-UCS pairings, a number of control procedures have
been designed. One of these is the *CS-alone control procedure*.
As Rescorla (1967) has indicated, the repeated CS-only presentations in this procedure test for sensitization. In the case of this
and other control procedures to be described, the "training trials"
are followed by a number of test trials. In effect, training trials
in the CS-alone control technique are identical to test trials because both consist of CS-only presentations. The standard forward conditioning procedure, to which experimental subjects may
be exposed, and the CS-alone control procedure are both illustrated in Figure 10.

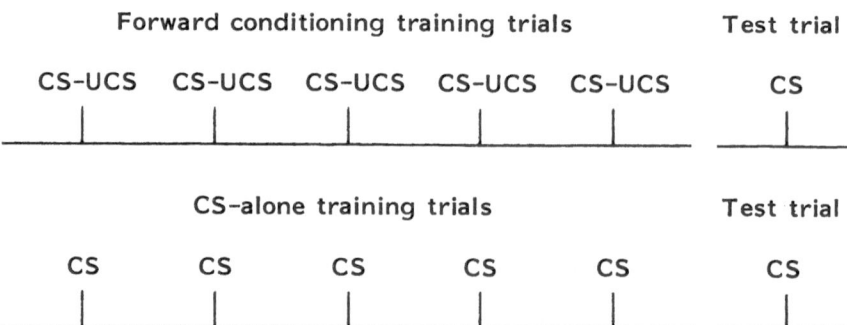

Figure 10. Forward conditioning procedure and CS-alone control
procedure.

A second procedure that has been used to control for the effects of Pavlovian conditioning is the *UCS-alone control procedure*. While experimental subjects receive the standard CS-UCS pairings during training trials, the control subjects in this procedure receive UCS-only presentations, as illustrated in Figure 11. This procedure is specifically designed to control for pseudoconditioning. If pseudoconditioning is observed in control subjects, the eliciting of a CR by experimental subjects cannot be attributed to previous training involving CS-UCS pairings.

Yet another classical conditioning control procedure, the *explicitly unpaired control*, has been described by Rescorla (1967). This method not only randomizes the separate presentations of the CS and UCS, but also equates the total amount of stimulation that is provided to the subject with that provided in the standard forward conditioning procedure. The amount of stimulation in either the CS-alone or UCS-alone control procedures obviously would not equal the amount of stimulation provided in forward conditioning where both CS and UCS are presented during training trials. Figure 12 illustrates the explicitly unpaired control procedure in which the CS and UCS are "never paired together in time" (Dunham, 1977, p. 75).

As mentioned earlier, *backward conditioning* may be used as a control procedure in classical conditioning experiments. The rationale for using this procedure as a control is that UCS-CS pairings should not produce associative learning. Therefore, if the CR occurred on a test trial following backward conditioning training trials, it would reflect the interference of nonassociative factors (Dunham, 1977). This control procedure is illustrated in Figure 13.

Dunham noted that if a specific CS-CR association has been learned during forward conditioning, the CR should reliably occur only to the CS that was originally paired with the UCS in Pavlovian conditioning trials. This rationale provides the basis for another control procedure called *discrimination control*. As illustra-

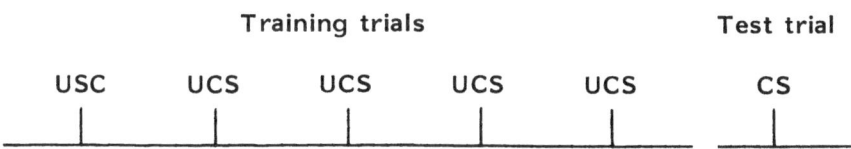

Figure 11. UCS-alone control procedure.

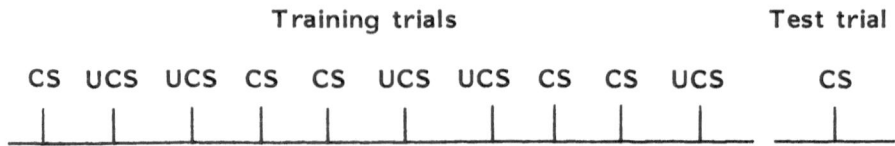

Figure 12.   Explicitly unpaired control procedure.

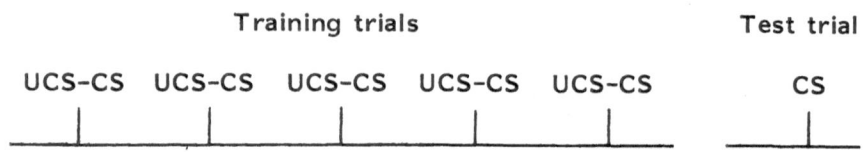

Figure 13.   Backward conditioning control procedure.

ted in Figure 14, one CS (CS_1) is always paired with the UCS but
another CS (CS_2) is presented in an explicitly unpaired manner.
If an association has been learned only between CS_1 and the UCS,
it would be expected that the CR would not be elicited by CS_2. If
the CR does occur to CS_2, it would be difficult to account for the
learning of this response on the basis of systematic CS_1-UCS pairings.

According to Rescorla (1967), there are problems with these
control procedures. For example, the explicitly unpaired procedure equates the total amount of stimulation presented to the
subject, but aside from this it does little more than eliminate
the CS-UCS forward pairing contingency during the training
trials. In fact, since pairings are not made, the presentation
of the CS actually indicates that the UCS will not be presented.
This in turn may lead to inhibition of the response when the

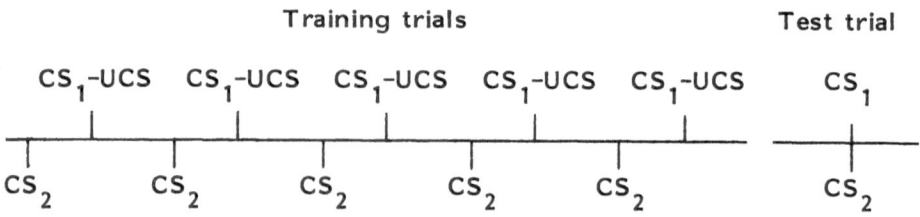

Figure 14.   Discrimination control procedure.

CS is presented. That is, the subject may learn a new contingency — that the CS is never followed closely in time by the UCS.
Another problem relates to the backward conditioning control procedure. Some researchers (e.g., McConaghy, 1971) have shown
that backward conditioning has produced results similar to forward conditioning when used in treating homosexuality.

Rescorla has devised a random control procedure that solves
the problems of the conventional procedures by eliminating any
contingency between the CS and the UCS. The two stimuli are
randomly programmed to include accidental or chance pairings. A
similarity may be noted between this procedure and the explicitly
unpaired control, but the primary difference is the inclusion of
accidental CS-UCS pairings which "eliminates the contingency. . .
[that] allows the CS to signal nonoccurrence of the US" (Rescorla,
1967, p. 74).

In a recent psychology of learning text, Schwartz (1978) has
schematically explained Rescorla's random control procedure in
three parts. The first two illustrations are not part of Rescorla's
procedure but Schwartz had included them in his schematization
to logically develop his discussion of Rescorla's model. First, he
described the standard pairing procedure in which a CS (e.g.,
tone) is paired with a UCS (e.g., shock), as illustrated in Figure
15. In this example involving a tone and shock, the shock *never*
occurs in the absence of the tone and the tone is *always* followed
by shock. In this way, a contingency exists between the CS and
UCS because the CS is a reliable predictor of the UCS. Conditioning should occur.

The second step in Schwartz's presentation of Rescorla's
method, illustrated in Figure 16, was a description of partial pairing. In this procedure, standard CS-UCS events are interspersed
among CS-only presentations. Although CS-UCS contiguity is
maintained by the CS-UCS pairings, the introduction of CS-only
presentations early in training weakens the contingency between

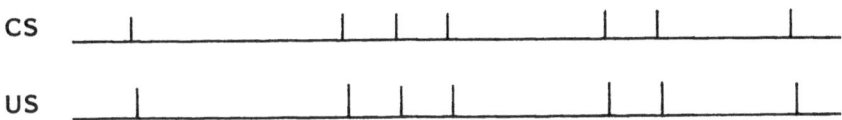

Figure 15. Standard pairing: p(UCS/CS) = 1.0, p(UCS/$\overline{CS}$ = 0.0.
From *Psychology of learning and behavior* by B. Schwartz. New
York: W. W. Norton, 1978, p. 86.

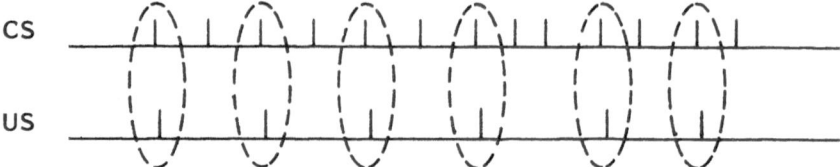

Figure 16. Partial pairing: p(UCS/CS) = 0.5, p(UCS/$\overline{CS}$) = 0.0.
From *Psychology of learning and behavior* by B. Schwartz. New
York: W. W. Norton, 1978, p. 86.

CS and UCS. This appears to contrast with standard conditioning
in which blocks of training trials, rather than single CS-UCS pairings, precede test trials. Although the CS in partial pairing cannot reliably predict the occurrence of the UCS as it could in the
standard pairing procedure, it nonetheless allows the subject to
accurately predict that the UCS will *never* be presented in the
absence of the CS. Minimal conditioning may be observed.

Schwartz's third illustration (Figure 17) depicts Rescorla's
random control procedure. In this procedure, the probability of
the UCS occurring in the *presence* of the CS is 0.5, as is the probability of the UCS occurring in the *absence* of the CS. In other
words, the UCS is just as likely to occur in the presence of the
CS as in the absence of the CS. No conditioning should occur in
this procedure because the contingency between CS and UCS has
been eliminated — that is, the CS provides no reliable information
about the occurrence or nonoccurrence of the UCS.

Despite findings by Rescorla (1968, 1969) that supported the
use of his random control procedure in classical conditioning experiments, recent investigations (Kremer and Kamin, 1971; Kremer, 1971; Quinsey, 1971; Benedict and Ayres, 1972) have shown
that some conditioning results from the accidental pairings of the
CS and UCS.

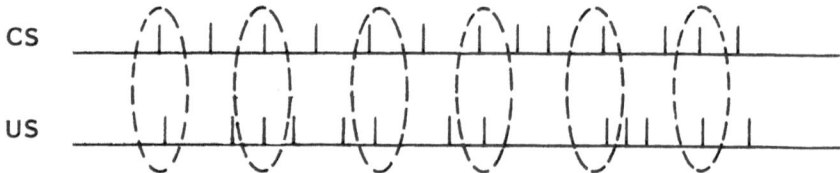

Figure 17. Random CS-UCS relation: p(UCS/CS) = p(UCS/$\overline{CS}$) =
0.5. From *Psychology of learning and behavior* by B. Schwartz.
New York: W. W. Norton, 1978, p. 86.

RESCORLA-WAGNER MODEL

The Rescorla-Wagner model mathematically illustrates the process by which CS-UCS associative strength increases with repeated presentations during Pavlovian conditioning trials (Schwartz, 1978). The model has been applied to the negatively accelerated learning curve that is typical for Pavlovian conditioning. According to the Rescorla-Wagner theory, the changes that occur in the magnitude of associative strength during training trials may be depicted as in Figure 18. Rescorla and Wagner have devised a formula to determine trial-by-trial changes in associative strength. These changes are mathematically expressed as a proportion of the difference between the asymptote (the maximum amount of

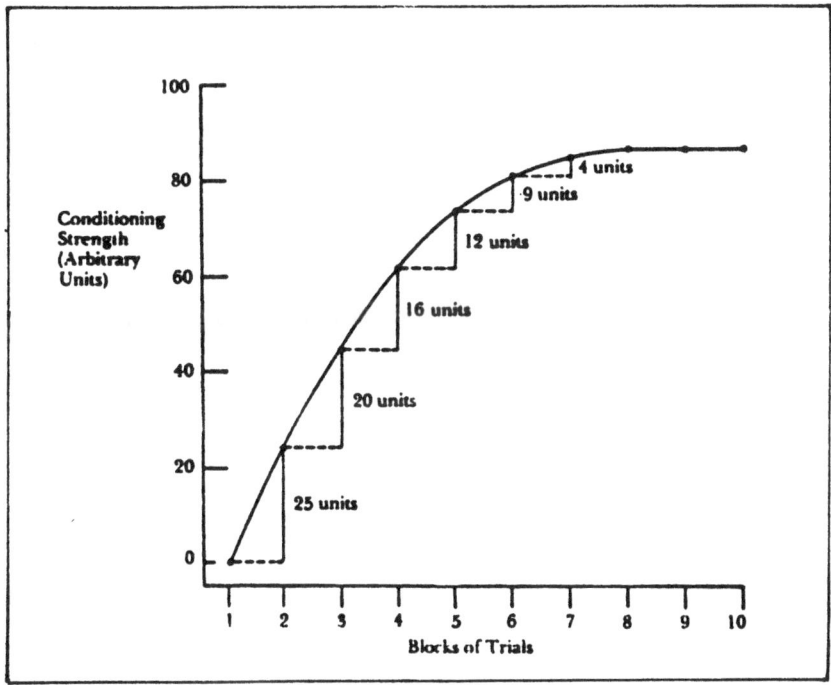

Figure 18. Idealized learning curve. The curve is negatively accelerated, which means that the amount of change in conditioning strength (in arbitrary units) gets smaller and smaller with repeated trials. From *Psychology of learning and behavior* by B. Schwartz. New York: W. W. Norton, 1978, p. 92.

learning) and the previous associative strength (previous level of learning). Their formula is $\Delta Vn = K(\lambda - V_{n-1})$, where V represent the cumulative associative strength and ΔVn the change in associative strength for any given trial. K is a constant value between 0 and 1 which, according to Schwartz, represents the observation that:

> Some CSs (the more salient ones) and some USs produce faster conditioning that other CSs and USs. Thus, the value of K influences the rate of conditioning (p. 93).

The symbol λ represents the asymptote, the level of which is determined by the nature and intensity of the UCS. The more intense a UCS, for example, the higher the leveling-off point of conditioning strength. Schwartz has provided an example of a hypothetical five-trial classical conditioning experiment to which the Rescorla-Wagner formula has been applied. In this example, $V = 0$, $K = 0.3$, and $\lambda = 90$ in Trial 1:

> Trial 1: $\Delta V_1 = 0.30(90-0)$ $= 27.0$
> Trial 2: $\Delta V_2 = 0.30(90-27)$ $= 18.9$
> Trial 3: $\Delta V_3 = 0.30(90-45.9)$ $= 13.2$
> Trial 4: $\Delta V_4 = 0.30(90-59.1)$ $= 9.3$
> Trial 5: $\Delta V_5 = 0.30(90-68.4)$ $= 6.5$

> Total associative strength after five trials = 74.9. (Schwartz, 1978, p. 94)

The progressively decreasing values of change (27.0 units of change on Trial 1; 6.5 units of change on Trial 5) during the increase in associative strength illustrates that less and less associative strength is contributed by each successive trial.

If the stimuli in a compound CS were equally salient, each stimulus should yield half the associative strength (Schwartz, 1978). If the tone in a tone-light CS were more salient than the light, however, it would be predicted that the associative strength of the tone would be greater than the associative strength of the light. In the following example, the K value for the tone is 0.7 while the K value for the light is 0.1, indicating that the tone is much more salient than the light:

$$\Delta V_{A(tone)} = K(\lambda - V_{AX}) \qquad \Delta V_{X(light)} = M(\lambda - V_{AX})$$

Trial 1:	$\Delta V_A = 0.70(90-0)$ $= 63.0$	$\Delta V_X = 0.10(90-0)$	$= 9.0$
Trial 2:	$\Delta V_A = 0.70(90-72)$ $= 12.6$	$\Delta V_X = 0.10(90-72)$	$= 1.8$
Trial 3:	$\Delta V_A = 0.70(90-86.4)$ $= 2.5$	$\Delta V_X = 0.10(90-86.4)$	$= 0.3$
Trial 4:	$\Delta V_A = 0.70(90-89.2)$ $= 0.6$	$\Delta V_X = 0.10(90-89.2)$	$= 0.1$

(Schwartz, 1978, p. 95)

This example demonstrates that the more salient stimulus in a compound CS has greater associative strength than the less salient
stimulus.

SECOND-ORDER CONDITIONING

As defined by Rescorla (1977), "second-order conditioning is
observed when a stimulus serves as a Pavlovian reinforcer only
by virtue of its own prior relation to the unconditioned stimulus"
(p. 135).

Holland and Rescorla (1975b) have demonstrated that second-
order conditioning is a more robust phenomenon than first-order
conditioning. Initially, rats were first- and second-order conditioned. After they were exposed to pairings of a food UCS and
illness-inducing rotation, responding to the first-order CS was
substantially reduced. There was little change, however, in the
rate of responding to the second-order CS. Restoring the value
of the food UCS increased responding to the first-order CS but
did not alter the animals' rate of responding to the second-order
CS. Hence, devaluation and subsequent increased evaluation of
a food UCS failed to affect the level of second-order responding.

The stability of a response to a second-order stimulus was
tested in another investigation by Holland and Rescorla (1975a).
After second-order conditioning was established in two groups of
rats, the response to the first-order CS was extinguished in one
of the groups. When tested for their response to the second-order
CS, subjects in both groups responded with the second-order CR.
The response to the second-order CS, therefore, was relatively
unaffected by changes in the response to the first-order CS.

Rescorla (1977) offered a plausible explanation for the finding
that second-order conditioning is more resistant to posttraining
manipulations than first-order conditioning:

> First-order conditioning apparently involves associations be-
> tween the CS and some representations of the US, because
> postconditioning changes in that US change the response to
> the first-order CS. However, many examples of second-order
> conditioning probably do not importantly involve associations
> with either of the obvious possible stimuli, the US or the
> first-order CS, because the current status of neither matters
> for the production of the second-order response. Instead,
> we have . . .argued that second-order conditioning may in-
> volve an association between the stimulus and the organism's

reaction to the first-order CS. The animal is presented with
a second-order CS, which is followed by a massive emotional
reaction; perhaps he learns the association between the two
(p. 158).

Rescorla's Second-Order Conditioning Procedures

Rescorla (1977) stressed that "the maintenance of a strong
response to the first-order CS" (p. 160) is the most important
condition for establishing second-order conditioning. Standard
procedures have involved pairing a CS (S1) with a UCS and subsequently pairing a second stimulus (S2) with S1 in the absence
of UCS presentations. A problem with this procedure is that first-
order conditioning rapidly extinguishes because of the removal
of the UCS at the time of S2-S1 pairings. Rescorla outlined two
procedures to minimize extinction of first-order conditioning and
to simultaneously prevent first-order conditioning to S2. The
first procedure involves the interspersing of S2-S1 pairings among
S1-UCS trials. An example is provided below:

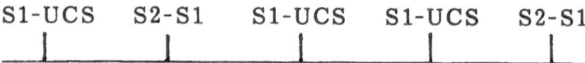

The second procedure employs an S2-S1-UCS sequence. The rationale is that if S1 is presented between S2 and the UCS, first-
order conditioning should occur between S1 and the UCS because
of their temporal closeness. In addition, the proximity of S1 to
S2 should produce second-order conditioning to S2. If the time
interval between S2 and the UCS is sufficiently long, first-order
conditioning should not occur between S2 and the UCS. In both
of Rescorla's procedures, the value of S1 appears not to be reduced as much as it would be in conventional Pavlovian second-
order conditioning.

Pavlovian Second-Order Conditioning in Instrumental Learning

Rescorla (1977) has argued that second-order conditioning
plays a major role in instrumental learning. The essence of his
hypothesis is outlined in the following excerpt from his 1977
study:

> Instrumental behaviors usually involve sequences of respon-
> ses, only the final member of which is actually coincident with
> the primary goal event . . . . It seems plausible to conclude
> that much of the responsibility for establishing incentive mo-
> tivation and learned reinforcement rests with higher-order

Pavlovian conditioning. To be sure, stimuli early in a sequence are often similar to those present at the final goal and consequently we can expect some of these properties to accrue to such stimuli by simple generalization. Additionally, however, they should gain their potencies by higher-order conditioning (p. 147).

Rescorla hypothesized that most behaviors in any instrumental sequence "should be supported by a mixture of first- and second-order Pavlovian conditioning" (p. 147). This being the case, behaviors furthest from the goal event should involve primarily higher-order conditioning and should be less affected by changes in the value of the goal event than behaviors nearest the goal. Hungry rats were trained to obtain food pellets by completing a maze of four successive T-units (Rescorla, 1977). The subjects were satiated to determine which aspects in the chain of instrumental responses would be maintained when the value of the goal event was changed. A systematic pattern was noted in the disruption caused by satiation. The response at the initial choice point was least affected, although at the end of acquisition training, this was the weakest component of the instrumental behavior sequence. Behaviors nearest the goal were most affected by satiation. Rescorla reasoned that the stimuli at the later choice points were the first to lose their effectiveness because they were directly followed by a first-order stimulus that was rendered ineffective by satiation. The consequence should be "a backward deterioration in performance under satiation" (Rescorla, 1977, p. 150). In further accounting for the stability of instrumental behaviors early in the free-operant chain, Rescorla discussed his observations in the light of Allport's functional autonomy theory of behavior. With respect to the role of this theory in second-order conditioning, Rescorla (1977) posited the following view:

Behaviors that become independent of their original goals may often do so because higher-order Pavlovian incentive motivation replaces the original motivation. As noted above, the power of higher-order conditioning for establishing motivation rests precisely on its apparent independence of the original motivations (p. 151).

HABITUATIVE AND ASSOCIATIVE FACTORS

Habituation was defined by Dodge as "the decrease and eventual disappearance of the reaction [to repetitive stimuli]" (Wyrwicka, 1972, p. 9). Similarly, Weisman (1977) referred to habitu-

ation as "the waning of behavioral, and electrophysiological, responses with repeated stimulation" (p. 3). The process of habituation may be "the result of a blockade in the sensory pathway
caused by the repetitive action of a stimulus" (Hernandez-Peon,
cited in Wyrwicka, 1972, p. 11). Reactions to most stimuli are
subject to habituation. The degree of habituation depends primarily on the intensity and the type of stimulus. According to
Wyrwicka, the higher the intensity of a stimulus, the lesser the
degree of habituation to it. Habituation occurs "more rapidly and
is deeper [greater] with weak stimuli such as tones than with sig-
nif[i]cant stimuli such as electric shock or food" (Wyrwicka, 1972,
p. 11), as illustrated in Figure 19. A typical illustration of habituation to electric shock was provided by Wyrwicka (1972). When
shock is applied to a dog's leg, the initial reaction is usually a
strong generalized motor response. After several shock trials,
the motor reaction becomes leg-specific and diminishes over the
course of a few days. If intensity and stimulus type are consid-

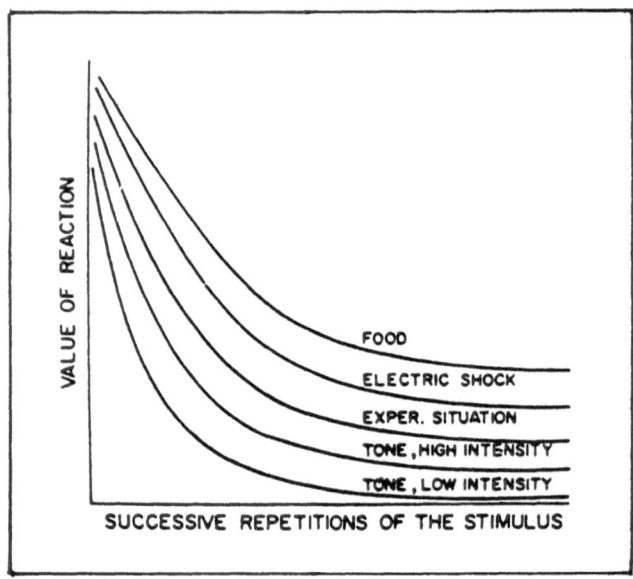

Figure 19. Possible effect of habituation on the value of reaction
to the repetitive action of various stimuli. From *The mechanisms
of conditioned behavior* by W. Wyrwicka. Springfield, Il.:
Charles C. Thomas, 1972, p. 11.

ered in combination, it follows that the response to a stimulus such as a weak tone would habituate more than the response to an intense tone; the degree of habituation to either tone would be greater than habituation to an appetitive or aversive stimulus. This, too, is illustrated in Figure 19.

Responses to complex stimuli have also been shown to habituate (Wyrwicka, 1972). For example, after several visits to a compartment, an animal gradually reduces its amount of exploratory behavior. It may actually cease its orienting-investigatory reaction, until such time as a new object is introduced to the compartment. At this point, the investigatory behavior is resumed but again gradually diminishes.

In his discussion of habituation, Weisman (1977) emphasized, as Wyrwicka (1972) had, that the degree of habituation depends on the nature of the stimulus. According to Weisman, habituation occurs at different rates to different stimuli depending on the motivational and biological relevance of the event. Differential habituation is significant to the learning of associations in Pavlovian conditioning because:

> It is likely that associations between neutral events and reinforcers endure with repetition, whereas associations between merely neutral events do not, in large part because of the differentially greater effect of the habituative processes on the latter events (Weisman, 1977, p. 4).

For this reason, the reinforcers used in Pavlovian conditioning are usually powerful, motivating stimuli that provide resistance to habituation.

Weisman proposed that supposedly learned behaviors are actually "learned modifications of innate behaviors" (p. 7). Consistent with this view, he has identified three mutually exclusive types of innate behavior that are often mistaken for highly purposive instrumental acts:

1. Orienting reactions — turning reflexes that allow the animal to locate himself with respect to the stimuli.
2. Basic locomotor activities — those activities that allow the animal to move from one location to another.
3. Action patterns — "preprogrammed complex behavioral units usually defined with reference to specific stimuli and deprivation states" (Weisman, 1977, p. 7).

The involvement of instinct conditioning in instrumental learning was not considered seriously until Brown and Jenkins (1968) discovered, in an autoshaping experiment, that a pigeon's key peck could be classically conditioned. This response was previously thought to be exclusively controlled by operant reinforcement. Schwartz (1978) has provided a typical example of autoshaping:

> Suppose we place hungry pigeons in a conditioning chamber and periodically present them with food. Suppose, in addition, that a few seconds prior to each food delivery, we light up a response key. Pigeons exposed to this kind of procedure reliably end up pecking just before food is delivered. In addition, they all end up pecking at the same place — the response key. This phenomenon has come to be called "autoshaping" (automatic shaping). Instead of training pigeons to peck a key, one can simply expose them to an autoshaping procedure (p. 320).

Weisman's (1977) account of the involvement of classical conditioning in autoshaping was that a biologically significant stimulus releases innate behaviors. In extending Weisman's proposition to Schwartz's illustration, it may be said that the food released the innate behaviors of orienting toward the lighted key, walking toward it (locomotor), and repeatedly pecking at the key (action pattern).

ENVIRONMENTAL AND COGNITIVE DETERMINANTS OF UCR AND CR

Weisman (1977) posited that UCRs and CRs are influenced by cognitive and environmental factors. First, with regard to UCRs, the behavior that is observed depends on the overlap between the organism's central representation of the reinforcer and the environmental conditions that elicit the response. Specific effects of environmental stimulation on the topography of the UCR were illustrated by von Holst and von Saint Paul (1963). In studying the effects of electrical brain stimulation and environmental models on the behavior of hens, von Holst and von Saint Paul (1963) found that without specific external environmental stimulation, the animal showed only generalized locomotor unrest. When brain stimulation was coupled with exposure to a closed fist, slight threatening actions were exhibited. When a stuffed polecat was presented in conjunction with brain stimulation, the hen vigorously attacked the stuffed animal. To determine the range of UCRs that can be elicited by stimulating a particular stimulus field in the brain, it seems necessary, therefore, to alter the environment in as many ways as possible. Second, Weisman (1977) described the cognitive and environmental determinants of the CR:

> When we say that an animal has learned the correlation be-
> tween one event and another, we may in cognitive terms mean
> only that the central representations of one event now include
> information about the other event. Thus, the neural corre-
> late of the CS becomes quite a cognitive structure, including
> considerable information about the reinforcer, its relationship
> in time to the CS, and probably at least some of its key phys-
> ical, biological, and emotional characteristics. When two
> events are correlated positively in time the result may be the
> construction of a second representation utilizing information
> available in the first. In classical conditioning this second
> representation should certainly resemble an animal's repre-
> sentation of the reinforcer, but it is unlikely to be the same,
> any more than a sketch drawn from memory is likely to be
> identical with one drawn from life. The central representa-
> tion, which evokes the UR, is constructed in the presence
> of the event itself, whereas the representation that evokes
> the CR is best viewed as a reinforcer memory, constructed
> only in the presence of information concerning the reinforcer
> encoded into the representation of the CS (p. 11).

CONSTRAINTS ON LEARNING

Pavlovian and operant conditioning procedures are not always effective in producing learning. Occasionally, conditioning does not occur or is observed to be only minimal despite the optimal correlation between CS and UCS in Pavlovian conditioning and R--S in instrumental conditioning. With respect to this problem, Black, Osborne, and Ristow (1977) have asserted that learning may be affected by system constraints. This type of constraint refers to "the limitations on change in a particular response that arise from the nature of the neural control system of which that response is a part" (Black et al., 1977, p. 38). According to these researchers, autonomic responses are especially sensitive to system constraints:

> There may be a limit on the amount of change that can be pro-
> duced as a function of the homeostatic feedback systems of
> which most autonomic responses are a component. The fact
> that . . . [it is difficult to obtain] decreases in heart rate
> below adaptation levels may be one example of this type of

constraint. Also, there may be system constraints that arise
from the relationship among different response systems. For
example, suppose that heart rate was linked to the system
controlling skeletal movement so that heart rate increases
could not occur unless skeletal movement occurred. We might
then limit the magnitude of conditioned heart rate increases
by requiring the subject to hold still during training and so
reveal a system constraint on the operant conditioning of
heart rate (Black et al., 1977, p. 38).

Weisman (1977) contended that learning may be hindered by
three types of constraints. One was the interference of highly
prepared instinctive responses with the learning of less prepared
operants. Several examples of this type of constraint were cited
by Breland and Breland (1961). In one instance, a raccoon was
trained to pick up a single coin. Next, the animal was required
to pick up a coin and put it into a container. Some difficulty was
experienced with the second task due to the interference of instinctive food-rubbing and washing behaviors. When required
to pick up two coins and place them in the container, the simula-
ted rubbing and washing behaviors interfered even more and prevented the animal from performing the task. Although not positively reinforced for the rubbing and washing ritual, the raccoon
nonetheless maintained this behavior.

A second constraint on learning, as indicated by Weisman
(1977), occurs when:

> The central representation of the response memory . . . is
> insufficient to enact the behavior. This may be because only
> stimulus aspects of the response are encoded, because the
> response is only part of an action pattern and has no separ-
> ate enactment code, or even because the aspect of the re-
> sponse for which selection is sought is not represented in
> memory (p. 18).

Third, constraints may be associative. In this respect, Weisman (1977) argued that:

> The response and the reinforcer may simply fail to be associ-
> ated even though they are, in fact, correlated. This seems
> an unlikely alternative; most responses are rich in stimulus
> properties to be associated with the reinforcer (p. 18).

Similarly, Black et al. (1977) have proposed that associative constraints interfere with classical and instrumental learning because
"certain stimuli, responses, and reinforcers are more likely to be

associated than others" (p. 38). Other writers (e.g., Seligman and Hager, 1972) have discussed associative learning in more detail.

PREPAREDNESS IN CLASSICAL CONDITIONING

The ease or difficulty of forming CS-UCS associations was discussed by Seligman and Hager (1972) in the light of the preparedness hypothesis. This hypothesis contrasts markedly with the equipotentiality hypothesis which asserts that:

Any natural phenomenon chosen at will may be converted into a conditioned stimulus . . . any visual stimulus, any desired sound, any odor, and the stimulation of any part of the skin (Pavlov, 1928, p. 86).

Because of the evolution of specialized sensory, response, and associative apparatus, it was Seligman and Hager's contention that an organism has certain predispositions in forming CS-UCS associations:

Not only may the CS be more or less perceptible to the animal and the US more or less evocative of a response, *but also the CS and US may be more or less associable* (Seligman and Hager, 1972, p. 4).

Hence, an organism will be either prepared, unprepared, or contraprepared to learn a particular contingency in a Pavlovian learning paradigm. These terms were meant to be used only in a relative sense because "nothing can be said to be absolutely prepared, unprepared, or contraprepared, but only more or less than something else" (Seligman and Hager, 1972, p. 5). To illustrate, Seligman and Hager cited a hypothetical experiment:

Suppose it takes a rat three pairings of the taste of licorice and apomorphine poisoning to show a full-blown aversion to licorice, and 129 pairings of licorice and foot shock for an aversion to develop, it would be inexact to say that the licorice-illness association was prepared and the licorice-shock association unprepared. Rather, the licorice-illness association was more prepared, or less unprepared, than the licorice-shock association (p. 5).

Interestingly, Seligman and Hager (1972) have noted that reports of human experiences support the preparedness hypothesis. To illustrate, they gave an account of how Seligman developed

taste aversion to a sauce subsequent to eating and becoming ill.
This sequence of events has been referred to as the Sauce Béarnaise phenomenon and may be schematized as follows:

Sauce Béarnaise - - - - Illness - - - - Vomiting
        CS   UCS   UCR

                                    - - Nauseating taste
                                              CR

Although Seligman's illness was attributed to the stomach flu and
not the ingestion of the sauce, and although the vomiting did not
occur until several hours after the meal, an aversion developed
to the taste of the sauce. These factors violated the laws of classical conditioning in several ways. First, classical conditioning
should not occur with long delays between the CS and the UCS.
Second, stimuli such as the other foods eaten during the meal,
the surroundings, and the people present should have become
aversive. Third, the process was not a cognitive one involving
expectations, as would be expected with classical conditioning;
that is, Seligman could not inhibit his aversion, even though he
knew that the sauce had not caused his illness.

     Evidence in the animal literature also favors long delay learn-
ing and the stimulus relevance concept. In an experiment by
Garcia, Kimeldorf, and Koelling (1955), rats acquired taste aversion to a sweet-tasting solution despite a time span of several
hours between the ingestion of the solution and the nauseating
effects caused by gamma radiation. It was not expected that an
association would be made between the taste stimulus and illness
because of the long interstimulus interval.

     The stimulus relevance phenomenon was demonstrated by Gar-
cia and Koelling (1972). Prior to the experiment, rats had demonstrated no preference for either tasty water or bright-noisy water. The tasty water was provided by adding flavors to the water
while bright-noisy water was provided by means of incandescent
lamps and a clicking relay. The rats were allowed to drink normal water or tasty, bright-noisy water in a second phase of the
experiment. Those who chose to drink the tasty, bright-noisy
water were exposed to x-ray radiation that produced nausea several hours later. In the final phase, the rats were given a choice
between tasty water and bright-noisy water. It was found that
an aversion developed to the taste stimuli but not to the audiovisual stimuli, which demonstrated that classical conditioning occurs more readily with some CSs and UCSs than with others.
Garcia and Koelling (1972) stated that the gustatory stimuli had

acquired secondary reinforcing properties which they termed
"conditioned nausea."

In another phase of the Garcia and Koelling experiment, a
second group of rats received shocks to the paws while drinking
the tasty, bright-noisy water. When later given the choice of
either tasty water or bright-noisy water, it was observed that
the rats avoided the bright-noisy water but drank the tasty water. Garcia and Koelling (1972) concluded:

> When shock which produces peripheral pain is the reinforcer,
> "conditioned fear" properties are more readily acquired by
> auditory and visual stimuli than by gustatory stimuli (p. 12).

On the basis of these two experimental manipulations involving
faradic shock and nausea-inducing UCSs, it may be stated that:

> (a) Rats tend to associate nausea with internal stimuli such
> as taste but *not* with external stimuli such as flashing lights
> and noises; and (b) rats tend to associate external pain stim-
> uli such as electric shock with external stimuli such as flash-
> ing lights and noises but *not* with taste stimuli (Dunham,
> 1977, p. 101).

The phenomena illustrated by the research of Garcia and his
associates may have implications for human research. If pictorial
or auditory stimuli are used in conjunction with an aversive stimulus to effect behavior change, faradic shock would appear to be
more appropriate than a chemical aversive stimulus. Conversely,
if the development of an aversion to taste stimuli is the intent of
the procedure, a chemical UCS may be more effective than an electrical UCS. These two assumptions were borne out in the empirical research of Lazarus (cited in Wilson and Davison, 1969, p.
328). Treatment of an alcoholic was unsuccessful when faradic
shock was employed as the UCS, but when a foul-smelling UCS
was used, alcohol consumption disappeared rapidly. Lazarus observed that:

> Faradic shock seems "appropriate" when the concern is with
> visual and/or tactile stimuli . . . [but] it may be inapprop-
> riate in handling overeating and alcoholic consumption (Wilson
> and Davison, 1969, p. 328).

Dunham (1977) has discussed four hypotheses that have been
advanced to account for delay learning and the stimulus relevance
phenomenon. The first was Seligman and Hager's preparedness
hypothesis which, according to Dunham, does not predict which
CS-UCS associations are readily transformed into CS-CR sequen-

ces. He asserted that this hypothesis merely describes the phenomena and "does not generate any testable predictions" (p. 103).
A similar criticism has been voiced by Rachlin (1970), who claimed
that the concept of preparedness cannot really be useful unless
it can "summarize some group of characteristics that prepared associations show and unprepared associations do not" (p. 170).
Long delay learning, for example, has not been found to be common "to all easily learned associations" and, therefore, until a
consistent set of rules can be established for all easily learned
associations, the concept of preparedness "will be limited in use-
fulness except as a synonym for ease of learning" (Rachlin, 1970,
p. 170).

Second, Dunham (1977) critiqued Garcia, McGowan, and
Green's (1972) formulation that evolution has provided certain
organisms with a nervous system that is predisposed to associate
olfactory and gustatory stimuli with visceral stimuli and to associate visual and auditory stimuli with cutaneous stimulation. They
further contended that:

> Since food absorption takes time, this system has become
> specialized to handle long interstimulus intervals (Garcia et
> al., 1972, p. 22).

Dunham (1977) claimed that this theory appeared to be limited in
generality. He partly based his criticism on the research of Wilcoxon, Dragoin, and Kral (1971) who observed that birds were
predisposed to associate visual and taste stimuli. This predisposition, however, may be species-specific and therefore does not
necessarily support Dunham's criticism of Garcia et al.'s hypothesis.

Third, the concurrent interference principle has been posited
by Revusky (1971) to account for delay learning and the stimulus
relevance phenomenon. According to Revusky, it is the interference of *relevant* stimuli during the interstimulus interval and not
the duration of the interval that disrupts an association between
two stimuli. With specific reference to the Garcia effect, Revusky
(1971) suggested that an association between taste stimuli and
nausea is learned because few relevant stimuli occur during the
interstimulus interval. Revusky called upon the biological predisposition notion to assist in categorizing stimuli that are relevant
and those that are not. For instance, if an organism is biologically predisposed to associate taste stimuli with illness, then stimuli
such as noise and lights that intervene during the interstimulus
interval would be *irrelevant* and should not interfere with associative learning. This principle is illustrated in Figure 20. Accord-

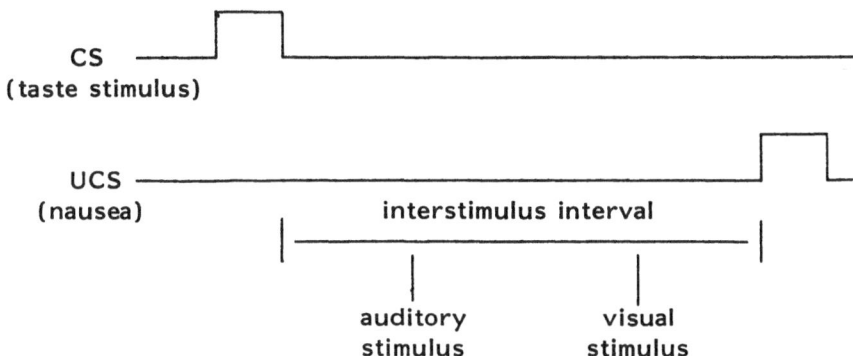

Figure 20. Irrelevant auditory and visual stimuli that do not interfere with taste-nausea associations. The auditory and visual stimuli are irrelevant because they are not of the gustatory class of
stimuli.

ing to the concurrent interference theory, taste stimuli that intervene during the CS-UCS interval interfere with the acquisition
of taste aversion and, therefore, may be regarded as relevant
stimuli. This is illustrated in Figure 21.

  Although Revusky's findings have supported the concurrent
interference proposition, Kalat and Rozin's (1971) research with

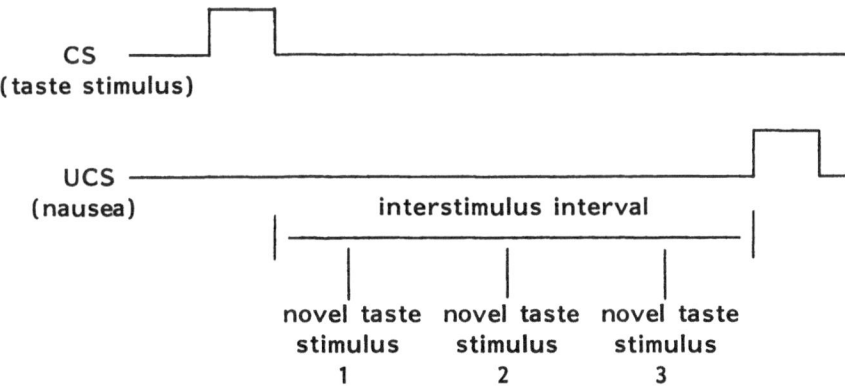

Figure 21. Relevant novel taste stimuli that interfere with taste-
nausea associations. Stimuli 1, 2, and 3 are relevant because, like
the CS, they are gustatory.

rats revealed that the formation of an association between a sweet solution and illness was not disrupted despite the introduction of three novel tastes in the 30-minute interval between the tasting of the sweet solution and the experience of illness. According to Dunham (1977), Revusky's account of delay learning and stimulus relevance is incomplete.

A fourth view is that of Mackintosh (1973), who claimed that an organism's lifetime correlations between tastes and nausea account for its ability to easily associate these types of events. The rat, for example, is predisposed to associate taste stimuli with nausea because of its exposure to an environment in which some flavors (poisons) have been repeatedly paired with nausea. Stated another way, if audiovisual stimuli in an organism's environment have *not* been associated with nausea, the organism may be unprepared (or even contraprepared) to form nausea CRs to audiovisual stimuli. According to Dunham (1977), the Mackintosh explanation seems to be a viable one that generates a number of testable predictions. Perhaps it would be possible to obtain entirely different results from those of the Garcia research if animals were reared in an environment in which auditory or visual stimuli were explicitly paired with nausea and in which taste-nausea associations occurred at random.

2
Aversive Control of Behavior: Paradigms and Research

Some behavioral problems, such as fears and compulsions, are under too much aversive control whereas positively motivated behavioral problems, such as alcoholism and sexual deviations, appear to be under too little aversive control. For the latter type of problems, aversion therapy techniques are most appropriate. *Aversion therapy* has been defined by Lovibond (1970) as a behaviorally oriented treatment that utilizes an aversive or noxious stimulus, such as faradic shock, to eliminate undesirable behaviors. Lovibond has defined an *aversive stimulus* as a "stimulus from which the subject will learn to escape, if given the opportunity" (p. 80).

EXPERIMENTAL PROCEDURES

Escape Learning

Escape learning is one of three common experimental procedures used in the aversive control of behavior. Specifically, a subject is presented with an aversive stimulus and is required to emit an appropriate response to escape from it. While human subjects can be given explicit directions for performing the instrumental escape response, animals must learn the response through trial and error. Lovibond (1970) has described a typical escape learning situation:

A rat is placed in a chamber with an electrifiable grid floor. When the shock is turned on, it stays on until the subject presses a bar on the side of the chamber. After a pause of

several minutes, the shock is again turned on. Characteristi-
cally, the subject may take a minute or longer to press the
bar on the first occasion. On successive trials, however, the
time taken to make the bar-press response, and turn off the
shock, decreases progressively until it approaches a minimum
of about a second (p. 81).

Lovibond stated that an escape response may not be necessary to
suppress undesirable behavior. He based his argument partly on
the work of Azrin (1960) who observed response suppression with
an aversive stimulus of 0.1 second duration or less. It is unlikely
that an escape response could have been made to a stimulus that
was presented for such a short time.

Hurwitz and Roberts (1977) identified several advantages of
escape learning procedures: (a) much guesswork about internal
processes is eliminated because the experimenter can unambiguous-
ly determine what the "stimulus to action was"; (b) the behavior
responsible for the offset of the aversive stimulus can be readily
observed; (c) relatively little variation is found in the data from
an escape learning experiment, as compared to a reward situation;
(d) "the criterion response cannot be construed as being part of
a decision-like process that would inevitably have led to the adop-
tion of a cognitive model" (p. 191).

Active Avoidance Training

A subject can learn to avoid, as well as escape from an aversive stimulus. In *active avoidance training*, a discriminative stimulus, such as a tone or a light, is presented prior to the onset of
the aversive stimulus. To avoid receiving the aversive stimulation, the subject must emit an appropriate response during the
presentation of the discriminative stimulus or before the onset of
the aversive stimulus. If the appropriate response is not made,
the aversive stimulus is administered to the subject (Hall, 1976).
Lovibond (1970) extended upon his example of escape learning involving shock and bar-pressing to illustrate active avoidance
training:

A buzzer is presented for 5-10 sec prior to shock onset and
continues with the shock . . . . If the subject presses the
bar before shock onset, the shock is prevented. Typically
the bar press comes under the control of the buzzer, and the
subject avoids the shock. The learned "behavior" is called
active avoidance because the subject must actively perform a
particular arbitrary response chosen by the experimenter in
order to avoid shock (p. 81).

Hall (1976) has likened the initial stages of avoidance training procedures to a classical conditioning paradigm:

> It should be recognized that during the early part of avoidance training, the procedure used mirrors a classical conditioning paradigm, since the organism has not learned to avoid the aversive stimulus (or UCS) and the UCS follows the signal (CS) in a fixed temporal relationship. It is only after some training trials have been provided and the subject learns to respond to the CS (thus avoiding the presentation of the UCS) that the "instrumental" aspects of the avoidance task are apparent (p. 191).

Passive Avoidance Training

A third procedure that may be employed in aversive control studies is *passive avoidance training*. Lovibond (1970) described the procedure as follows:

> The subject is first trained to perform some instrumental act for positive reinforcement; for example, pressing a bar for food, or running along a short runway to drink. When the instrumental act is well established, its performance is followed by aversive stimulation. That is to say, the subject is now shocked when it presses the bar or runs to the water bottle. The avoidance "behavior" which follows the application of aversive stimulation is called *passive avoidance* because the subject avoids the aversive stimulus if it simply refrains from carrying out the positively motivated act (p. 81).

Lovibond drew attention to a similarity between passive avoidance learning and operant punishment. He claimed that these operations were similar because they both involve:

> [A] procedure whereby aversive stimulation is made contingent upon the performance of the response to be eliminated (p. 82).

Aversion-relief

A relief stimulus is often used as an adjunct to escape and avoidance procedures in the aversive control of behavior. In an *aversion-relief procedure*, a deviant stimulus is paired with an aversive UCS while a positive alternative stimulus is associated with UCS offset. The subject can either terminate or avoid the aversive stimulus by emitting the appropriate escape or avoidance response, respectively. The underlying assumption of aversion-relief is that:

> Any stimulus that is present during the termination of an aversive stimulus will come to have a positive valence: that is, it will be accompanied by feelings of "relief" (Rimm and Masters, 1974, p. 369).

This type of procedure, therefore, is designed primarily to "influence subsequent behavior by reducing the attractiveness of problem behaviors and stimuli and increasing the attractiveness of alternative, acceptable behaviors and stimuli" (Rimm and Masters, 1974, p. 377). Rimm and Masters have described aversion-relief in terms of escape and avoidance:

> Initially, aversion relief is actually an escape procedure, and after this technique has been employed for several treatment sessions, or trials, a client may be allowed to *avoid* the aversive stimulus by requesting or otherwise self-administering the termination of the display of inappropriate stimuli and the onset of the relief stimuli *before* the punishing event has occurred. For example, after the inappropriate stimuli are displayed, the client may have 8 seconds before a shock will occur, during which time he can terminate the display, institute the display of more appropriate items, and in doing so avoid the shock (p. 371).

The aversion-relief component of escape and avoidance training is clearly illustrated in Feldman and MacCulloch's (1965) treatment of homosexual behavior. Subjects were permitted to escape shock by pressing a switch to replace a slide of a nude male with a slide of a nude female. They subsequently learned to avoid the shock by pressing the switch prior to the scheduled onset of the aversive stimulus.

A cogent description of the aversion-relief procedure has been provided by Kanfer and Phillips (1970):

> The method of an aversion-relief combination . . . offers an incompatible response as an alternative to the UCS. The "relief" portion of treatment utilizes a desirable response as a potential positive reinforcing stimulus, deriving its positive qualities from its contiguity with aversion-escape. Theoretically, either the anxiety associated with the CS-UCS interval is reduced . . . or positive emotional responses are conditioned to termination of the noxious UCS . . . . The relief

stimulus thus is intended to accomplish two functions: (1) it
serves to provide an avoidance or escape response, and (2)
it increases the potential reinforcing property of the associated stimulus event, . . . The practice of the desirable response, coupled with the probable explicit or implicit social
approval from the experimenter and the provision of an alter-
nate response, may . . . yield important practical benefits in
therapy (pp. 344-345).

Although not schematized by Kanfer and Phillips (1970) nor by
Rimm and Masters (1974), the aversion-relief procedure can perhaps be depicted as in Figure 22.

Rimm and Masters (1974) emphasized that not only should the
inappropriate stimulus be paired with the aversive stimulus, but
so should any "remaining image of the stimulus" (p. 370). Hence,
the aversive stimulus "should be continued for a while after the
[pictorial] stimulus is no longer visible" (p. 370). This procedural manipulation may be especially important in aversion therapies incorporating instrumental escape. If an instrumental response is used to simultaneously terminate the aversive stimulus
and the stimulus representing the undesirable behavior, then any
images about the deviant stimulus that remain after the escape response is made will be associated with the relief effects of aversive stimulus offset. Figure 23 represents the sequence of events
that occur when the termination of the aversive stimulus coincides
with the offset of a deviant pictorial stimulus. In this illustration,

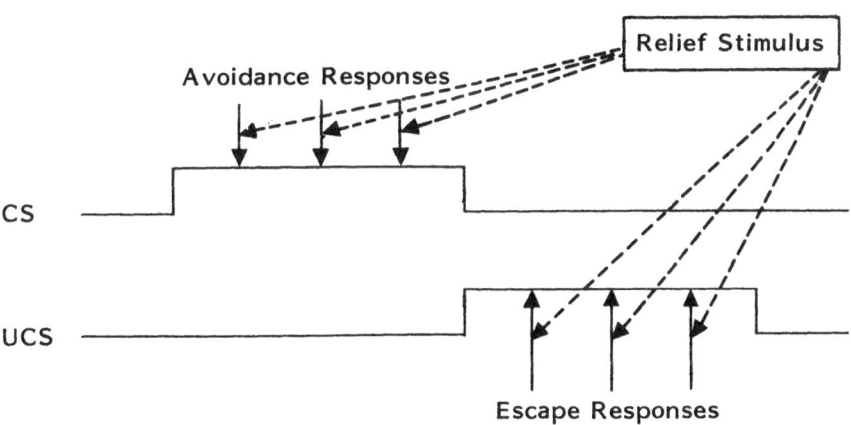

Figure 22. Escape and avoidance paradigms employing a relief
stimulus.

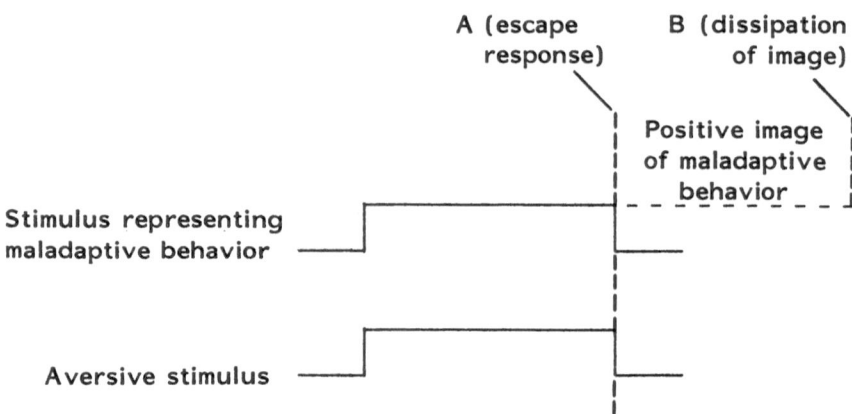

Figure 23. Treatment paradigm in which an instrumental escape response simultaneously terminates the aversive stimulus and the deviant pictorial stimulus.

A represents the point at which the aversive stimulus and the maladaptive behavior stimulus are terminated simultaneously by an instrumental button-press response. Thereafter, the subject's inner behavior (represented by A-B time interval), which may involve positive fantasies about the undesired behavior, is positively reinforced because of its association with relief from the aversive stimulus. In Figure 24, A represents the point at which only the deviant stimulus is terminated by the subject's instrumental response. The aversive stimulus is continued so that during the A-B time interval, the subject's positive imagery about the deviant stimulus is paired with the aversive stimulus. Point B represents the dissipation of the imagery and the termination of the aversive stimulus. Extending the aversive stimulus to point B minimizes the possibility of an association between the deviant imagery and aversion relief. Although the formulation may be accurate, the problem remains of ascertaining precisely how long the UCS should continue after the instrumental escape response has been made.

Delaying the offset of the aversive stimulus has been found by several researchers (Bolles and Warren, 1966; Leitenberg, 1965b; Lovibond, 1963) to not weaken the effectiveness of the noxious stimulus in suppressing undesirable behaviors. These

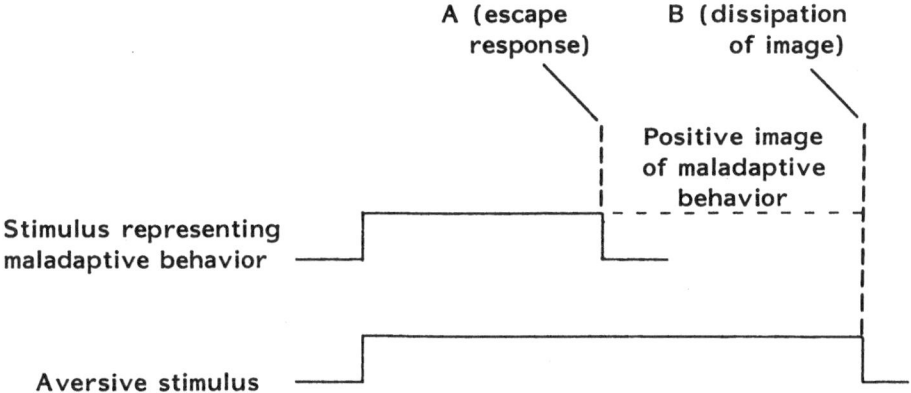

Figure 24. Treatment paradigm in which the aversive stimulus continues for a designated time after the deviant pictorial stimulus is terminated by an instrumental escape response.

findings provide some support for Rimm and Masters' recommendation to delay the offset of the aversive stimulus in aversion-relief procedures. It is recognized, however, that these findings do not relate directly to Rimm and Masters' rationale for continuing the aversive stimulus, and that the studies involved response-contingent-aversive-stimulation.

OPERANT–PAVLOVIAN INTERACTIONS IN
AVERSION THERAPY

Both instrumental and classical conditioning may be involved in aversive control procedures. Mikulas (1978) has succinctly delineated the instrumental and classical components of aversion therapy by making a crucial distinction between aversive counterconditioning and operant punishment:

Aversive counterconditioning . . . is based on respondent conditioning, the systematic pairing of two sets of stimuli, one which elicits the undesired response and one which elicits the aversion response. The stimuli are paired independent of what responses the client makes. The client's responses are only a measure of the progress of the conditioning. Operant

> punishment . . . is based on operant conditioning. Here the
> aversive stimulus is presented contingent upon a particular
> response of the client and usually occurs if and only if the
> client makes the response. Consider the use of an unplea-
> sant odor in the treatment of over-eating. In aversive coun-
> terconditioning, the odor would be paired with cues that tend
> to elicit or encourage over-eating, as a way of weakening the
> support for over-eating. In operant punishment, the odor
> would be paired with the response of over-eating as a way to
> suppress the act of over-eating (p. 65).

A similar if not identical view was expressed by Moss, Rada, and
Appel (1970):

> The aversive . . . [stimulus] can be paired either with a
> stimulus secondarily associated with the undesirable behavior,
> or with the behavior itself. When paired with a second stim-
> ulus, the paradigm is generally a respondent (Pavlovian) one;
> when paired with the undesirable behavior, the paradigm is
> generally an operant (Skinnerian) one (p. 291).

While the classical and instrumental components of aversion
therapy may be operationally differentiated, their effects are difficult to separate. Bandura (1969) asserted that instrumental conditioning often produces some classical conditioning effects:

> When a given behavior is punished, stimuli arising from the
> punished response itself, and environmental events present
> at the time, may become endowed with negative properties
> (p. 502).

On the other hand, because a UCS may reinforce any behaviors
that occur during the CS-UCS interval, responses may be operantly conditioned within a Pavlovian conditioning procedure. Even
the classic study by Watson and Rayner (1920) in which a fear response was conditioned in an 11-month-old child has been regarded by Church (1966) as an example of instrumental, not classical,
conditioning. It has been generally reported that this experiment
used classical conditioning procedures, since a conditioned fear
response to a rat was produced by pairing the presentation of the
rat (CS) with a loud noise (UCS). Church (1966) claimed, however, that the procedure involved instrumental conditioning on the
basis of two points. First, the aversive UCS was administered
contingent on Albert's response of touching the rat and not merely on the presence of the rat. [Note: In their laboratory notes,
Watson and Rayner (1964) did indeed report that "just as his hand

touched the animal the bar was struck immediately behind his head" (p. 22).] Second, it was reported that the UCS was not presented if Albert put his thumb in his mouth when the CS was presented.

The problem of separating the effects of instrumental and classical conditioning was further illustrated by Rachman and Teasdale (1969), who questioned Feldman and MacCulloch's contention that the effectiveness of their therapy for homosexuals was due primarily to operant-type anticipatory avoidance conditioning. Rachman and Teasdale's argument was that classical conditioning was an integral part of Feldman and MacCulloch's anticipatory avoidance procedures. Shock was delivered on "one-third of the trials whether the patient . . . [made] a button pressing response or not" (Rachman and Teasdale, 1969, p. 296). In other words, on one-third of the trials, there was no provision for escape from or avoidance of the aversive stimulus. These trials were Pavlovian conditioning trials. Rachman and Teasdale proposed, therefore, that the program was effective because of the classical conditioning of anxiety to homosexual stimuli.

Lovibond (1970) questioned the use of the term classical conditioning to describe the aversion therapy of sexual deviations. He believed that the procedures only remotely resemble those used in classical conditioning laboratory experiments. Lovibond commented that:

> Experimental literature on classical conditioning relates to those forms of behavioral modification in which a *previously indifferent* or neutral stimulus is given signal significance through pairing with an . . . unconditioned stimulus. In aversion therapy of sexual deviations, however, a stimulus (usually visual or verbal) which evokes a positive sexual response is followed by aversive stimulation in the hope of suppressing the sexual response to that stimulus. Clearly, this is a special case of punishment [R → S or sexual arousal → punishment?], and it can scarcely be taken for granted that the findings from experiments on classical conditioning of neutral stimuli may be transferred directly to the treatment situation (p. 87).

ESCAPE LEARNING: THEORY AND RESEARCH

The feasibility of studying animal behavior has made it possible to obtain detailed information about the characteristics of escape behavior. Although it may be difficult to generalize some of the information to human studies, such a review is nonetheless a valuable prerequisite to the study of human escape behavior involving a lever- or button-press response. In analyzing the behavior of rats in lever-press escape learning, Davis (1977) identified two aspects of the response to be learned. One was the topographical component (freezing), and the other was the location of the response (on the lever). Hence, freezing on the lever would be the appropriate escape response. The topography and location of responses that may occur during lever-press escape training are summarized in Figure 25. An animal's initial responses in escape training were considered by Bolles (1970) to be natural responses to aversive stimulation and were termed SSDRs (species-specific defense reactions). When rats were used as subjects, Bolles and McGillis (1968) proposed that SSDRs involved exploratory movement when the animals were initially placed in the experimental chamber, followed by a scrambling attempt to escape upon the onset of shock. According to Bolles and McGillis, the response of pressing on the lever is made accidentally while the rat is attempting to escape. This response not only terminates the shock but results in the rat remaining "frozen" on the lever, as represented by cell A of Figure 25. The responses that are recorded by the experimenter are, according to Bolles and McGillis, merely reflexes to shock onset or current-induced muscular con-

| | Response | |
	Freezing	Other behaviors
Lever	(A)	B
Other areas of the cage	C	D

Figure 25. Topography and location of responses in lever-press escape training. Adapted from "Response Characteristics and Control During Lever-press Escape" by H. Davis. In H. Davis and H. M. B. Hurwitz (eds.), *Operant-Pavlovian interactions*, Hillsdale, N. J.: Lawrence Erlbaum, 1977, p. 239.

tractions that cause the lever to be released momentarily and
hence allow for a subsequent depression of the lever. Competing
SSDRs, such as fleeing or fighting (Figure 25, matrix cell B) are
very unlikely to result in the acquisition of a consistent lever-
press (Bolles, 1970). It is also unlikely that the freezing response will occur in areas where the lever is not located (cell C)
because of the essential role of the lever in terminating the shock.
Freezing responses in other areas of the cage are punished by the
continuous presence of shock and therefore are not likely to be
maintained. Cell D of Figure 25 represents behaviors other than
freezing (fighting or fleeing) in areas other than the one in which
the lever is located. This is the most unlikely combination of behaviors to occur during training.

Pavlovian Analysis of Lever-Press Escape Behavior

While Davis (1977) has analyzed lever-press escape on the
basis of SSDRs, the systematic presentations of shock in his procedure led him to consider a Pavlovian analysis. Although no external CS was presented, it is possible, according to Davis, that
some aspect of the cage environment gained control over SSDRs
and functioned as a CS. Davis also proposed that the SSDRs elicited by the hostile environment (UCS) may be regarded as UCRs.
With repeated exposure, a selected response in the SSDR hierarchy (freezing on the lever) becomes the CR. Therefore, the
"transition from general to specific, in terms of both the environment and the subject's behavior, may represent the transition
from unconditioned to conditioned elements" (Davis, 1977, p. 243).
A Pavlovian analysis of escape behavior, however, was not entirely satisfactory to Davis because:

> It retains the "terror" inherent in SSDRs but shifts its source
> from the general US to specific features of a CS . . . . Simi-
> larly, the focusing on freezing from the SSDR hierarchy does
> not suggest that the role of "fear", per se, has been reduced.
> We would therefore prefer to see the effects of increased ex-
> posure to the situation reflected in a gradual reduction of
> "fear" or "terror", not in a change in the stimuli that caused
> them (p. 243).

Measurement of Lever-Press Escape Behavior

Davis (1977) and his colleagues have recently devised a computerized technique to record the duration, time of occurrence,
and fluctuations in the force of lever contact during lever-press

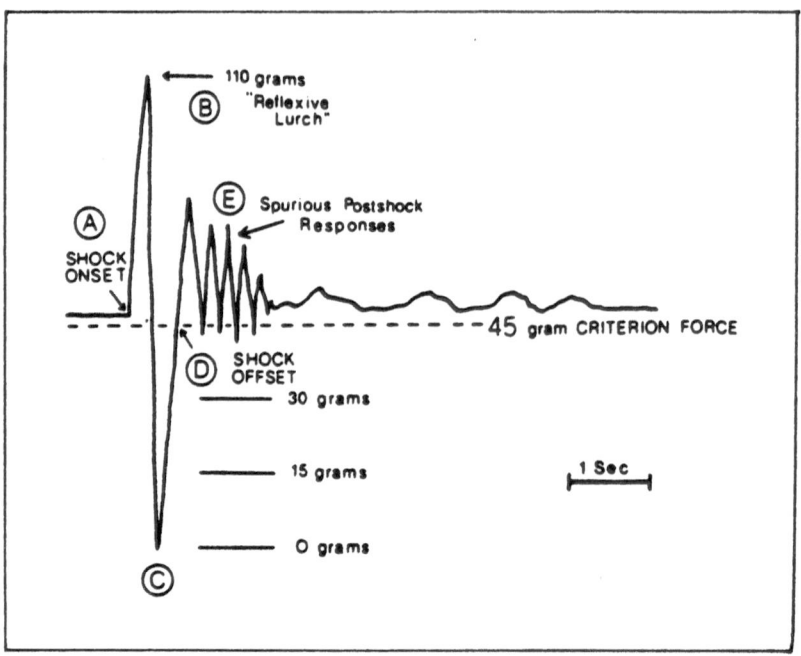

Figure 26. Composite illustration of the essential features of lever contact during the initial portion of a lever-press escape trial. From "Response Characteristics and Control During Lever-Press Escape," by H. Davis. In H. Davis and H. M. B. Hurwitz (Eds.), *Operant-Pavlovian interactions*, Hillsdale, N.J.: Lawrence Erlbaum, 1977, p. 251.

escape training. Figure 26 illustrates the major characteristics of the pattern that this technique detected in the force and stability of lever contact behavior. In elaborating on these essential features of lever contact, Davis (1977) explained:

> Prior to shock onset the subject was in contact with the lever at approximately 48-gm force. Immediately following shock onset (Point A), a reflexive lurch, which appears on virtually all escape records, occurs (Point B). This appears on the lever contact record as a brief spike of peak force, typically in excess of 100 gm and occasionally reaching values above 150 gm. As a consequence, the subject is briefly out of contact with the lever, during which time the force record returns to 0 gm (Point C). The subject typically returns to

contact with the lever rather quickly, which appears as a rapid increase in force followed by a short period of erratic contact. As the rapidly increasing force first passes from 0 through the criterion value, a "response" is recorded and shock is terminated (Point D). This entire portion of the sequence typically occurs in less than one-half second. The brief period of erratic force that follows shock offset may result in a spurious "discrete" response count (Point E) if the force values associated with lever contact are centered near the criterion . . . . Relatively minor shifts in posture may result in responses being recorded each time the force of lever contact drops below and again passes through criterion . . . . The force of lever contact for the remainder of the intertrial interval is typically quite constant, varying as little as 5 gm for the remaining 25-sec period (pp. 250-252).

Computerized recording has two advantages over conventional discrete response measurement:

1. As illustrated by Point E in Figure 26, Davis' technique can detect changes in force that are below the force value of the reflexive lurch and that are produced by (a) "metabolic activity (respiration) of a subject that was otherwise motionless on the lever while 'anticipating' shock" and by (b) postshock response bursts (Davis, 1977, p. 253).

2. Whereas Davis' method enabled the recording of *all* on-lever behaviors, apparatus of the fixed-criterion type is insensitive to on-lever behavior that occurs below the criterion force value. This means that if the criterion value is changed, the subject's behavior may be misinterpreted as having changed in frequency. Raising the criterion value may result in fewer responses being recorded, while lowering the criterion value may give the impression of increased frequency of responding (Davis, 1977).

SSDR vs. Instrumental Lever-Press Response

Davis, Hirschorn, and Hurwitz (1973) attempted to measure the freezing response independently of the lever-press response. For one group of rats, escape from shock was contingent on a response that lifted the lever while subjects in another group escaped by pressing on the lever. Davis et al. found that escape response latencies did not differ between the two groups. The

amount of time spent in freezing on the lever after escape responses were made, however, was significantly lower for the lever-
lift subjects than for the lever-press subjects. The subjects in
the lever-press group spent a mean of 85.5% of the training session holding the lever, while subjects in the lever-lift group held
the lever for only 6.5% of session time. The majority of lever-lift
subjects, however, assumed an immobile freezing position under
the lever between escape responses. A freezing response, therefore, was a dominant feature in escape behavior for both groups.
Davis (1977) interpreted this finding as providing support for the
SSDR analysis of escape behavior.

The results of a study by Davis and Kenney (1975) illustrated
that differences in test chamber design affect escape response
topography. Subjects in the Lehigh Valley chamber performed a
cyclic routine of holding the lever between shock presentations,
lurching off briefly at shock onset, and immediately pressing the
lever to terminate the shock. Subjects trained in Campden cham-
bers, however, were observed to leap forward from the mid-cage
area at shock onset, make a discrete lever-press response, and
return to the mid-cage area. The Campden subjects initially tried
but abandoned the "lever holding-reflexive lurch strategy" (Davis, 1977, p. 245) because the position of the lever made this strategy awkward. The naturalness with which the lever-holding response was emitted, even by the subjects in the Campden chamber, supports SSDR theory.

When Lehigh Valley subjects were transferred to the Campden
chamber in a second phase of the experiment, their continuous
lever-holding was reduced to 30% of session time. The subjects
who spent approximately 8% of session time in lever-holding in the
Campden chamber during Phase I increased their lever-holding
to only 15% of session time when transferred to the Lehigh Valley
chamber.

SSDR-Operant Analysis of Lever-Press Escape Behavior

Davis (1977) stressed that the low-latency responses that occurred early in escape training were essentially reflexive in nature and could not be viewed as discrete aversively maintained
operant responses. In furthering his analysis of lever-press escape behavior, however, Davis proposed that at some point during
training, there is "a shift in the basis of control from SSDR to
operant reinforcement" (p. 240). The observation that the topography of the escape response remains essentially the same
throughout training makes it difficult to identify this critical

transition point. Davis' computerized recording technique, however, is very sensitive to variations in lever contact force and
thereby may more accurately identify the point of transition from
SSDR to operant control. On the basis of several investigations
(Davis and Burton, 1974; Davis, Porter, Burton, and Levine,
1976), Davis (1977) concluded:

> 'Pure' SSDRs, that is, the "raw terror" of freezing, is more
> likely to result in a "heavy-handed" lever press than is the
> lever-holding behavior of a subject that has become reason-
> ably "relaxed" in the escape situation and is now under con-
> trol of the escape reinforcement contingency (p. 255).

Specifically, these studies revealed that:

> The mean force of lever contact recorded over the first three
> escape sessions appeared . . . to be considerably higher in
> force (averages ranging from 75 to 93 gm) than in later ses-
> sions (averages typically declining to near 40 gm) (p. 255).

In summary, it appears that behavior during the early stages of
escape training may be adequately explained by SSDR theory
while the operant conditioning model more appropriately accounts
for escape behavior later in training.

PREDICTABLE VS. UNPREDICTABLE
AVERSIVE STIMULATION

Subject preference for predictable or unpredictable aversive
stimulation was discussed by Seligman and Binik (1977) in terms
of (a) the preparatory response proposition, (b) the safety signal
hypothesis, and (c) the uncertainty reduction hypothesis. Seligman and Binik considered the presence of a stimulus that reliably
predicts the *nonoccurrence* of an aversive event to be "the fundamental psychological event that limits fear" (p. 166). They called
such a stimulus a safety signal. In his publication, *Helplessness:
On depression, development, and death*, Seligman (1975) provided
a cogent description of the safety signal hypothesis:

> When traumatic events are predictable, the absence of the
> traumatic event is also predictable — by the absence of the
> predictor of the trauma. When traumatic events are unpre-
> dictable, however, safety is also unpredictable: no event re-
> liably tells you that the trauma will not occur and that you
> can relax (p. 112).

Seligman illustrated a number of ways in which safety signals operate in the natural environment. For example, he wrote that in the bombings of London during the Second World War:

> Each [air] raid was predicted by sirens some minutes in duration. When no sirens were on, Londoners carried on admirably, without undue tension and in good cheer (p. 113).

It was argued by Seligman and Binik (1977) that when an aversive stimulus is used in classical conditioning, the presence of the CS (absence of the safety signal) increases the subject's fear while the absence of the CS (presence of the safety signal) reduces the subject's fear. If there were no CS to reliably predict the occurrence of the aversive UCS, then the subject would be in chronic fear.

The uncertainty reduction hypothesis, advanced by Berlyne (1960), is similar to the safety signal hypothesis in its predictions but it may be applied to both aversive and appetitive UCSs and to neutral stimuli. According to this proposition, the reduced uncertainty that accompanies predictable UCS onset is the basis for subject preference for predictable UCSs. The uncertainty reduction hypothesis appears not to incorporate the fear notion for aversive UCSs, as does the safety signal hypothesis, but it is nonetheless conceivable that uncertainty about the onset of an unpredictable aversive stimulus may contribute to chronic fear.

Perkins' (1955) preparatory response hypothesis also proposes that predictable UCSs are preferable to unpredictable UCSs. The presentation of the CS would enable the subject to make a response that could reduce the discomfort produced by an aversive UCS. This hypothesis, like the uncertainty reduction proposition, neglects the aspect of fear in predicting a preference for predictable aversive events.

Preference for predictable shock has not always been a consistent finding in studies involving human subjects. Badia, Suter, and Lewis (1967) found only a weak preference for predictable shock among undergraduate university students. The subjects were tested in an inescapable shock situation to determine (a) whether they preferred warned or unwarned shock, and (b) if warned shock were preferred, whether it was due to the information provided by the CS or to the opportunity that the CS provided for making a preparatory response. In the Badia et al. (1967) study, subjects selected either signalled or unsignalled shock on each trial. Shock was signalled if the subject chose to receive signalled shock and, conversely, the shock was unsignalled if the subject indicated unsignalled shock as his preference.

Two groups of subjects participated in the study. One group received shock on 100% of the trials and a second group received shock on only 25% of the trials. Subjects in both groups were informed that their choices would in no way affect the number of shocks they received. Although the subjects in the 25% group did not receive shock on each trial, they nonetheless were required to indicate on every trial whether they preferred signalled or unsignalled shock. For this group, there were two uncertainties with regard to the presentation of shock: (a) the trials on which the shock would be presented, and (b) the precise time of shock onset. For the group that received shock on every trial, there was only one uncertainty — the precise time of shock onset.

The preparatory response hypothesis predicts that subjects in both the 100% and 25% groups would prefer signalled shock because "preparation is a function of the signal and not the amount of information it provides" (Badia et al., 1967, p. 272). The uncertainty reduction hypothesis predicts, however, that more subjects in the 25% group would prefer signalled shock. In other words, preference for signalled shock would be greater as shock uncertainty increases. This prediction was supported by the finding that in the 25% condition, significantly more subjects indicated a preference for warned shock. Preference for warned shock did not develop in the 100% shock group.

The reasons given by the subjects for preferring signalled shock were threefold. First, they could relax until CS onset. Second, they could prepare for the shock by becoming alert, sitting up straight, or by tensing up. Third, they felt the shock was weaker when preceded by a warning. Subjects who preferred unsignalled shock said they did so because their thoughts during the no-shock intervals were not interrupted by signals. Also, the signals made them tense and anxious. Some reported that the shock felt more intense when preceded by a warning and others stated that, with the signal, it was like getting shocked twice.

Pervin (1963) investigated three variables of the certainty-uncertainty dimension — signal, no signal, and inconsistent signal. In addition, the effect of two independent variables in a control-helplessness dimension were studied, i.e., subject shock control and experimenter shock control. Male undergraduate students indicated that for the certainty-uncertainty dimension, their order of preference was signal, inconsistent signal, and no signal. From the first to the third session, however, signalled shock became "less preferable and more anxiety-arousing while . . . [unpredictable shock] became more preferable and less anxiety-arousing" (Pervin, 1963, p. 583). According to Pervin, predictability

is preferred in novel, threatening situations whereas some degree
of uncertainty is preferred under repetitive, nonthreatening circumstances. Subjects reported that they preferred signalled
shock for basically three reasons. First, they could prepare psy-
chologically for the shock by developing an attitude of acceptance
toward it. Second, they could prepare physically for the shock
by bracing their leg, to which the electrodes were attached.
Third, they could rest during the safety signal interval and think
of things other than the shock. In view of these reasons, perhaps the preference for predictable shock in Pervin's experiment
can best be explained in terms of the preparatory response and
safety signal hypotheses.

With regard to the control-helplessness dimension, the results
revealed that subject shock control was clearly preferable to experimenter control. In this respect, Pervin (1963) wrote:

> The basis of the preference for, and anxiety-reducing pro-
> perties of, control is not entirely clear. It may be suggested
> that in this experiment interpretation of the S-control situa-
> tion as one of mastery cued off relief in connection with past
> experiences wherein mastery prevented trauma. In relation
> to this, control may provide hope for the eventual influenc-
> ing of the stimulus itself. Beyond these factors, control may
> satisfy a basic or culturally induced need for mastery (p.
> 582).

Several investigators (Averill and Rosenn, 1972; Geer, 1968;
Glass and Singer, 1972) have studied the specific effects of predictable and unpredictable aversive stimulation on the galvanic
skin response in humans. In these studies, GSRs were measured
during intershock intervals for unpredictable shock subjects and
during the safety period between UCS offset and CS onset for
subjects in a predictable shock condition. The similarity between
these two intervals is the absence of both a CS and UCS. A between-groups comparison of the GSR measures revealed that subjects in the unpredictable shock group showed more arousal than
the subjects in the predictable shock group. In other words,
more arousal was experienced when no stimulus was available to
predict the onset of the aversive event. Although increased
arousal does not necessarily indicate increased fear, the difference in GSRs between the two groups can perhaps be interpreted
as being functionally related to safety signals.

Safety signal function has also been investigated with infra-
humans. Badia and Culbertson (1970) found that when rats were
required to make a bar-press response to escape shock, subjects

in the unpredictable shock group spent more time holding the bar between escape responses than subjects in the predictable shock group. This finding is consistent with the prediction of the safety signal hypothesis that unpredictable shock engenders more fear than predictable shock. Such an interpretation can only be made, however, if it is assumed that fear was the motivating factor in bar-holding behavior.

Seligman (1968) and Seligman and Meyer (1970) found that rats exposed to unpredictable shock developed more ulcers than those exposed to predictable shock. Again, the safety signal notion is supported if "more ulcers reflect more fear" (Seligman and Binik, 1977, p. 170). Seligman and Binik (1977) cautioned, however, that the differences in ulceration findings may have been artifactually amplified by differences in the amount of food consumed by the animals. The subjects in the unpredictable shock group bar-pressed less frequently than the predictable shock subjects and consequently received less food. Having less food in their stomachs than the subjects in the predictable shock group may have made them more susceptible to ulcers.

Seligman and Binik (1977) pointed out that although there is considerable evidence to support the safety signal hypothesis, it has both empirical and logical problems. One empirical problem concerns a frequently used measure of stress — weight loss. On the basis of the safety signal hypothesis, weight loss should be greater in subjects who have been exposed to unpredictable shock. Research findings have not been consistent with this prediction. Weight loss is often greater or not different for subjects in predictable shock conditions than for unpredictable shock subjects (Brady and Esty, 1963; Friedman and Ader, 1965; Weiss, 1970, 1971). The finding by Bowers (1971) that human subjects had a lower heart rate when they could not predict the onset of shock than when shock onset was predictable presents another empirical problem. According to the safety signal notion, heart rate should be accelerated during unpredictable shock because of increased fear.

One logical problem for the safety signal hypothesis is the difficulty of determining the intensity of fear. The accuracy of the prediction that there is less fear during predictable shock than during unpredictable shock cannot be determined unless the magnitude of fear can be measured in each case. Although the total time spent experiencing fear is less during predictable shock, it remains to be determined if the intensity of fear differs between the two shock conditions. Another question concerning the logic of the safety signal hypothesis was posed by Seligman and Binik (1977):

Why [should] a stimulus paired with unpredictable shock produce chronic fear as opposed to chronic relief? . . . If the
background stimuli in an unpredictable shock situation co-oc-
cur with shock onset, offset, and absence, why do the fear-
evoking properties of shock onset become conditioned instead
of the relief properties of offset and absence? (p. 176).

Seligman and Binik were not completely satisfied with their explanation but, nonetheless, they asserted that:

Animals happen to be built that way. It makes evolutionary
sense that in a situation in which noxious events occur un-
predictably, animals remain in fear until they find a reliable
predictor of safety instead of remaining complacent until they
find a more reliable predictor of danger (p. 176).

CHARACTERISTICS OF AN EFFECTIVE
AVERSIVE STIMULUS

Nonspecific arousal can be maintained by uncertainty. In the
case of aversion therapy, uncertainty may be increased by "varying the intensity, duration, time of onset, and site of action of
the aversive stimulus . . . . [and] by introducing intermittency
into the reinforcement schedule" (Lovibond, 1970, p. 85). Lovibond contended that the major effect of increasing uncertainty
would be to reduce the "perceptual disparity between training and
extinction conditions" (p. 86) which serves to increase the resistance of a response to extinction. According to Lovibond, therefore, uncertainty associated with an aversive stimulus increases
its effectiveness. Kushner (1970) has discussed the positive features of a faradic stimulus:

1. The most desirable feature of a faradic stimulus is that
    it can be easily administered. While technicians can be
    readily trained to operate a faradic shock apparatus,
    highly skilled medical personnel should be present when
    nausea-inducing drugs are used.
2. A faradic stimulus produces virtually no side effects. If
    the apparatus is safely designed and if subjects are
    screened for heart conditions, the use of a faradic shock
    stimulus should not be hazardous. Drugs, on the other
    hand, may cause serious side effects.
3. Faradic stimulation is experienced immediately upon being
    administered, whereas the nauseating effects of a chemi-
    cal aversive stimulus may be delayed. In addition, the

effects of a faradic stimulus are reasonably predictable,
whereas reactions to an emetic vary from individual to individual, and even from treatment to treatment for the
same subject. For these reasons, a faradic shock stimulus "permits much better control and accurate presentation of CS-UCS and response-shock temporal sequences"
(Kushner, 1970, p. 29).

4. A faradic stimulus permits the therapist to administer a
    stimulus of precise intensity for a precise duration of time
    at precisely the required moment. A chemical stimulus
    does not have these advantages.

5. A faradic stimulus can be varied over a wide range of val-
    ues which permits the study of the effects of differing in-
    tensities of aversive stimulation on the magnitude of re-
    sponse suppression.

6. The problem of relapses is easier to deal with if a faradic
    rather than a chemical aversive stimulus is used. The
    use of booster treatments and intermittent reinforcement
    can be more readily programmed with a faradic stimulus.

Faradic shock is very effective as an aversive stimulus in situations in which certain behaviors, such as self-injury, must be
immediately eliminated (Rimm and Masters, 1974). Mildly aversive
procedures may be inappropriate in such instances because of the
time they require to eliminate the behavior. Rimm and Masters
(1974) referred to a study by Bucher and Lovaas in which only
four treatment sessions and 12 shocks were required to eliminate
head-banging behavior in a 7-year-old psychotic boy. The same
behavior was eliminated in a psychotic girl "after a total of only
15 contingent shocks" (p. 379). Another illustration in the Rimm
and Masters discussion was Risley's successful treatment of a 6-
year-old girl for dangerous climbing activities. With home-based
treatment by means of a portable shocker, it was found that "within 4 days, climbing at home was reduced from 20 to an average of
2 instances a day, and within a few weeks it disappeared entirely"
(Rimm and Masters, 1974, p. 380). The finding not only illustrated the effectiveness of faradic aversion therapy[1] in treating behavior requiring immediate cessation but also the adaptability of

---

[1]According to Logan and Turnage (1975), faradic aversion therapy refers to "the application of an electrical aversive stimulus to
some portion of a subject's or patient's extremity (generally),
with the ultimate goal of eliminating some specific (*continued*)

faradic aversion techniques to the home environment. According to Rimm and Masters (1974), two additional points favor the use of a faradic stimulus: (a) the behavior to be treated need not be one over which the individual has voluntary control and (b) treatment need not be restricted to adults. With respect to the first point, Rimm and Masters cited a study by Sachs and Mayhall in which "the incidence of spasms and involuntary movements in a cerebral palsied individual [was reduced] from more than 100 per hour to the low rate of 6 per hour" (p. 381). The effectiveness of faradic stimulation in treating children is supported by a number of studies. For example, Lang and Melamed (1969) eliminated ruminative vomiting in a 9-month-old infant and Galbraith, Byrick, and Rutledge (1970) eliminated the same problem in a 13-year-old retarded boy.

A faradic shock stimulus has the added advantage that it can be administered by means of a portable apparatus. In this way, an individual can self-administer the aversive stimulus contingent on his emitting the deviant response in the natural environment. It is even possible to design an apparatus that *automatically* delivers the aversive stimulus upon each occurrence of the undesired response. Such an adaptation of a portable stimulus shocker has been illustrated by Scholander (1972). This researcher provided an interesting description of a light, portable, and easily-handled apparatus that was designed to treat a 14-year-old epileptic boy's habit of gripping his neck with his hands. One electrode was enclosed in a bracelet worn around the wrist and the other was located in a coil on the patient's shoulder. When the individual's hand approached to within a predetermined distance of his neck, an electronic relay was activated and a shock was delivered to his wrist. The patient's neck-gripping behavior was eliminated in 1 month, and after 9 months he was still free of his habit.

There is little information on the optimal magnitude of electrical stimulation needed to produce an effective aversive stimulus because researchers usually do not report sufficient detail. Reports tend to involve qualitative statements to the effect that the level of shock was either subjectively calibrated or determined on

---

(*Footnote continued*)
maladaptive behavior(s)" (p.33). This term is preferred by Logan and Turnage (1975) to the traditional term 'electrical aversion therapy' so as to distinguish this type of aversion therapy from electroshock therapy.

the basis of unpleasantness felt by the experimenter. For instance, in treating an infant's ruminative vomiting, Lang and Melamed (1969) used an intensity of shock that the therapist judged
to be painful and to which the infant showed distress. The guideline used by Feldman and MacCulloch (1965) was to raise the intensity level of the faradic stimulus until the subject reported it
to be "more unpleasant than he . . . [found] the CS (e.g., a male
stimulus) to be pleasant." They added that the level of shock
"should vary randomly about the level described by the patient
as being unpleasant" (p. 167). In the Vogler, Lunde, Johnson,
and Martin (1970) research into faradic shock conditioning of
chronic alcoholics, the "initial shock intensity was set at about 3
milliamps, subjectively reported to be painful" (p. 303). Adjust-
ments were made, however, for subjects "who were seemingly unaffected by this level of shock intensity, or who appeared to be
adapting to it" (p. 303).

An interesting finding reported by Berecz (1972) was that females self-administered lower shock intensities than males. Subjects were required to "self-administer 15 shocks during each session, and to record the intensity levels employed" (p. 245). Berecz also reported that "self-administered shock intensities increased both within a given session, and across the sessions as
a whole" (p. 245).

In treating a transvestite by response-contingent aversive
stimulation, Moss et al. (1970) monitored the subject's reactions
to faradic stimulation and adjusted shock intensity accordingly.
They stated:

Although the initial shock level was reported by the patient
as mildly painful, as treatment progressed habituation occurred, and the level was raised (Moss et al., 1970, p. 292).

Pervin (1963) determined the maximum endurable shock level in
human subjects by gradually increasing the intensity of the shock.
Pervin observed that there was a progressive adaptation to the
level of shock during experimental sessions. To keep the shock
intensity at the maximum endurable level, Pervin regularly increased the intensity prior to each session. Although not reported, the 'operational measure' of maximum endurable shock presumably was the subject's indication that he could not tolerate a
higher level.

Because details about a faradic shock stimulus are not always
indicated in published accounts of aversion therapy studies, Butterfield (1975) has recommended that the following information
should be reported:

(1) The type of shocking device used. (2) Its output characteristics — (a) voltage output when applied to the patient;
(b) the current path through the patient; (c) wave form and
polarity of current; (d) current amplitude; (e) the frequency
of the current; (f) the duration of the application. (3) The
electrode sites. (4) Electrode design and material. (5) Electrode area. (6) Type and amount of electrode paste, if used.
(7) The response-shock stimulus relationships, (e.g., how
soon after response occurs does the shock start and how long
after the response stops does the shock continue). (8) In
the case of classical conditioning procedures the CS-UCS relationship should be specified. (9) Other special procedures,
if used (p. 107).

PROBLEMS AND ETHICAL ISSUES

There are conflicting views concerning the optimal level of
anxiety required for effective chemical or faradic aversion therapy. While Bancroft recommended that "a high level of anxiety
is necessary for successful treatment," Eysenck and Rachman
claimed that "highly anxious patients may respond unfavorably to
aversion treatment" (in Rachman and Teasdale, 1969, p. 283).
Turner and Solomon's guideline for using aversion therapy with
highly anxious subjects was that:

A highly emotional subject will proceed most rapidly if we
start off with a short CS-UCS interval and then lengthen it,
at the same time that we start with an intense UCS level then
lower it to produce longer latency escape responses. When
these procedures are combined, we should be able to produce
rapid learning (cited in Rachman and Teasdale, 1969, p. 286).

As indicated by Rachman and Teasdale (1969), the guideline proposed by Turner and Solomon does not align with "Azrin and
Holz's (1966) view that the UCS intensity should not be altered"
(p. 287).

In the case of faradic aversion therapy, fear of shocks may
increase an individual's anxiety level and interfere with the development of conditioned responses. If the intensity of the shock
is too high and generates too much anxiety, some patients may be
reluctant to continue with therapy. If the intensity is too low,
counterconditioning of the inappropriate behavior may not be ac-
complished. Rimm and Masters (1974) stressed that although

physical harm should be avoided, a faradic stimulus should be administered at the maximum intensity that the client can endure.

At least one writer (Wolpe, 1958) has specifically used mild
levels of shock to *inhibit* human anxiety. The therapeutic method
developed by Wolpe was based on the research of Mowrer and
Viek. These researchers exposed two groups of rats to continuous electrical stimulation and observed that:

> Those animals which were able to learn a definite motor re-
> sponse (jumping into the air) as a precursor to the termina-
> tion of the shock soon lost their anxiety at being placed in
> the experimental cage *minus* the shock, whereas animals
> given exactly the same amount of shock without the oppor-
> tunity to learn a specific motor response did not tend to lose
> their anxiety at all (Wolpe, 1958, pp. 173-174).

On the basis of these observations, Wolpe postulated that motor
responses may be advantageously used in treating human anxiety:

> If in the presence of a stimulus evoking neurotic anxiety a
> mild shock were repeatedly to be applied to the limb of the
> patient, and if this shock were also each time to produce a
> well-defined motor response, the neurotic anxiety would grad-
> ually be weakened (p. 174).

Wolpe (1969) postulated that repetition of the stimulation would
lead to "conditioned inhibition of the autonomic responses that are
evoked at the same time" (p. 159). Wolpe (1958) successfully
treated a severe case of agoraphobia by this technique. The procedure used in treating a 23-year-old female agoraphobic is summarized in the following excerpt:

> She was instructed to close her eyes and imagine a relatively
> easy (though to her, slightly disturbing) fall and to signal
> at the beginning of the imagined movement. At this signal
> a mild electric shock (secondary of Palmer inductorium at 8.0
> cm with a 6-volt dry cell in primary) was passed into her
> forearm, being stopped only upon the occurrence of a brisk
> flexion of the forearm, which the patient had been instructed
> to make. This movement soon became the instant response to
> the shock. She found that the shock was not uncomfortable
> (as it would be at other times) and the *shock-cum-flexion* "van-
> quished" the disturbed feeling. When the whole sequence had
> been repeated a number of times (usually between 15 and 40),
> she reported that imagining the fall was becoming less unplea-
> sant and disturbing and, after further repetitions, that she

could imagine it with ease. Thereafter she was able to attempt this particular fall in actuality and, after practicing it a good many times a day, could do it easily after a few days. Then she was ready for a slightly more difficult fall (Wolpe, 1958, pp. 176-177).

Personal communication with J. Wolpe clarified whether or not the motor response of flexing the forearm functioned as an escape response:

The well defined motor response was not conceived to function as an escape response, but as a response competitive with anxiety, parallel to the findings of the Mowrer and Viek experiment. The shock was quite mild and certainly not what could be called aversive . . . . Perhaps the competition with anxiety was due to the intruding sensory stimulus and the motor response may have played no part at all (Wolpe, personal communication).

Wolpe's finding related to the use of mild shock intensities to inhibit anxiety might well be considered in determining the level of shock to be used in aversion therapy. If mild shocks have been found to reduce anxiety, it seems to follow that intense shocks would increase anxiety. This formulation tends to be consistent with the views of Bancroft and Rimm and Masters.

Rimm and Masters mention three additional problems for aversion therapy. First, if provision is not made for acquiring alternative acceptable behaviors, the "next behavior in the individual's personal hierarchy may appear, and this behavior may not be appropriate either" (Rimm and Masters, 1974, p. 366). A second problem is behavioral rigidity − that is, the desired behavior may be successfully developed to the extent that "it becomes a rigid part of the person's repertoire and may not be replaced, temporarily or permanently, by different behaviors when they are more appropriate" (pp. 365-366). To illustrate, Rimm and Masters asserted that if a child is punished for sexual exploratory behavior, he may at a later time "find himself impotent, inhibited, or simply unmotivated toward appropriate sexual encounters" (p. 366). The use of aversive techniques may give rise to a third problem; namely, "the acquisition, by the client, of various skills and predilections for personally administering similar aversive stimuli to others" (Rimm and Masters, 1974, p. 367). They added that this problem was more likely to occur "when children are involved and when the modification procedures occur in a naturalistic environment such as the home" (p. 367).

Bandura (1969) cautioned that stimuli to be associated with an aversive stimulus should be distinctive and delimited so that "needless aversions and avoidance behaviors" can be minimized (p. 509). The aversive stimulus should be potent enough to effect the desired behavior change but at the same time it must confine generalization to a particular class of activities. Inappropriate generalization can be regulated by differential reinforcement procedures whereby "undesirable events are repeatedly associated with negative experiences, while the desired ones are paired with either rewarding or no adverse consequences" (Bandura, 1969, p. 510). In addition, the technique of verbal labelling may be used to delimit and enhance the most relevant aspects of the stimuli to be negatively conditioned. In this procedure, the presentation of the deviant stimulus is supplemented by verbal descriptions of the client's related deviant activities. This information may be provided by the therapist or may be recorded in the client's own voice.

A criticism that has often been levied against aversion therapy procedures is that they are inherently inhumane. Rimm and Masters (1974) contended, however, that:

Many therapists . . . feel that a minimal number of mild shocks is more humane than the continual, but ineffective, spanking or shaming of a child. Often this may also be the case in instances requiring the use of more powerful aversive stimuli . . . . Many individuals feel that . . . physical debilitation and the prolonged use of strait jackets or practices such as tying a self-destructive child's feet and arms to his bed are more morally reprehensible than the application of short-term procedures of aversive control (p. 381).

In addition, long-term restraint procedures may lead to "demineralization of bones, shortening of tendons, and an increasing loss of movement ability" (Rimm and Masters, 1974, p. 363).

According to Rimm and Masters, aversive techniques are also advantageous in gaining control over behaviors that are both highly rewarding and physically or mentally harmful. Problems such as drug abuse, for example, may require "the manipulation of extremely aversive consequences if they are to be brought under control" (pp. 363-364). The rapid control of behavior that is possible with aversive procedures, therefore, constitutes an important ethical consideration for these types of behaviors.

Moss et al. (1970) claimed that "a behaviorally-oriented alternative to aversion therapy does exist and can be effective in cases as resistant to treatment as sexual deviations" (p. 294).

These researchers employed both response-contingent aversion
therapy and positive behavioral control procedures in treating two
transvestites. The aversion therapy client received randomly
presented shocks to the upper part of his back while cross-dressing. The shock was discontinued when the client began to remove the female clothing. In this procedure, shock functioned as
"both a punishment for cross-dressing and as a discriminative
stimulus for undressing, i.e., escape" (Moss et al., 1970, p. 292).
The subject in the behavioral control condition was instructed to
limit his transvestite activities to a specific set of stimuli, i.e., to
cross-dress only in the storage room of his house. He was also
instructed to keep a record of the frequency and duration of the
occasions on which he cross-dressed in addition to a cumulative
record of the number of days on which he did not cross-dress.
These records provided feedback about the progress of therapy
and may also have functioned as an incentive for the client to
dress appropriately. For both subjects, cross-dressing was reduced to zero, although the results were more immediate with
aversive control. With this procedure, cross-dressing was eliminated after the first session, whereas with the stimulus control
procedure, 6 weeks were required to eliminate the deviant behavior. The subject that had been treated by positive reinforcement
and stimulus control, however, reported complete abstinence from
the deviant behavior during monthly posttreatment follow-up in-
quiries conducted over 8 months. The aversion therapy subject
failed to return beyond the first follow-up visit.

For some behaviors, "symbolic, or imagined, representations
of the behavior or of the stimuli that elicit the problem behavior
. . . [are the] items to which aversive procedures are applied"
(Rimm and Masters, 1974, p. 372). For example, a homosexual
may be sexually aroused by the mere thought of a nude male.
Hence, homosexual responses may be counterconditioned by pairing an aversive stimulus with either pictorial presentations of
nude males or verbal descriptions related to homosexual stimuli.
Also, symbolic or imagined negative consequences may be used in
place of a faradic or chemical stimulus. The use of either real or
symbolic stimuli in therapy are dictated not only by the nature of
the problem behavior but also by practical constraints and ethical
considerations.

Rimm and Masters (1974) recognized that aversion therapy
"will always involve the infliction of pain, physical or mental" and
that "mere approval by a client for the use of aversive techniques
does not immediately justify them" (p. 362). The following state-

ment by these writers on the issue of justification undoubtedly reflects the outlook of many behavior therapists:

The only true justification for the eventual use of aversive procedures is the likelihood that they will be effective in changing a person's behavior in the desired direction, leaving no residual ill effects, again either physical or mental (Rimm and Masters, 1974, p. 362).

PAIN THRESHOLD AND PAIN TOLERANCE

Rogers and Vilkin (1978) investigated diurnal variation in sensory and pain thresholds for cutaneous electrical stimulation and changes in these thresholds with mood states. The subjects were young male and female hospital workers and medical students, each of whom had volunteered to participate in the study. Subjects were instructed to make two verbal responses:

(1) "Now" (i.e., ascending detection threshold) as soon as the subject begins to feel the slightest amount of any kind of sensation of electricity.

(2) "Pain" (i.e., ascending pain threshold) as the first sensation changes into any kind of pain, ache, or hurting sensation (Rogers and Vilkin, 1978, p. 431).

The two thresholds and mood state were evaluated in the morning and in the evening on 6 separate days. There was a significantly higher mean detection threshold in the morning than in the evening. As indicated by Rogers and Vilkin (1978):

The mean value for the A.M. was 1.66 milliamperes with a standard deviation of 0.55 while the mean value for the P.M. was 1.46 milliamperes with a standard deviation of 0.57 (p. 432).

The morning values for pain thresholds were also significantly higher than the evening values:

The mean value for the A.M. was 6.22 milliamperes with a standard deviation of 2.85. The mean value for the P.M. was 5.61 milliamperes with a standard deviation of 2.77 (Rogers and Vilkin, 1978, p. 432).

Rogers and Vilkin indicated that there were (a) no significant correlations between "states of happiness, fatigue, anger, depression, activity and fear and the detection and pain thresholds"

(p. 432); and (b) no "significant variation in mood states between morning and early evening" (p. 438).

Glynn and Lloyd (1976) investigated diurnal variation in the subjective ratings of pain of pathological origin. The main purposes of their study were:

(1)   To determine whether there was a diurnal variation in the intensity of pain reported.

(2)   To determine whether the nature of the diurnal variation in pain, if found, differed for patients in terms of . . . personality type, age, sex . . . [etc.].

(3)   To determine whether the intensity of the pain reported was related to subjective alertness (Glynn and Lloyd, 1976, p. 370).

Patients with intractable pain reported their subjective alertness and the intensity of their pain every 2 hours between 8:00 a.m. and 10:00 p.m. for 7 days. Both ratings were made on visual analogue scales.

Glynn and Lloyd found that reported intensity of pain increased in a nearly linear fashion throughout the day, excepting slight peaks at mid-day and 6:00 p.m. They noted that this trend was similar to the trend in diurnal variation in pricking pain found in a study by Procacci (in Glynn and Lloyd, 1976). One striking difference, however, was the time of day at which the maximum intensity of pain was reported. In Procacci's study, it was 6:00 p.m., whereas in Glynn and Lloyd's study, it was 10:00 p.m., the last recording of the day.

Although the *shape* of the diurnal variation graph in Glynn and Lloyd's study was similar for males and females, females reported more intense pain. They also showed a rise in reported intensity throughout the day that was "three times as large as that for males" (p. 370). These findings could be interpreted to mean that females are more sensitive to pain than males and that their subjective feelings of pain rise more rapidly from morning to evening.

Using data from the same subjects, Glynn and Lloyd (1976) found a significant difference in the reported intensity of pain between subjects who remained at home during the day and those who were employed. Two trends were outlined:

The reported pain of those who stayed at home rose rapidly from 08.00 to 12.00 and then remained relatively constant over the rest of the day. In contrast, the reported pain of those patients who went out to work decreased from 08.00 to

10.00 and remained below the 08.00 level until shortly after 16.00. It is interesting to note that the reported pain of this latter group was considerably lower than that of the patients who stayed at home, even in the evening, when both groups were presumably at home (Glynn and Lloyd, 1976, p. 371).

In the same study, diurnal variation in pain differed significantly between introverts and extroverts. This finding is amplified in the following statement:

Introverts reported rather more pain than extroverts between the hours of 10.00 and 14.00 but approximately the same amount at the other times of the day (p. 371).

A significant difference in the diurnal variation of pain was also found between neurotic and stable individuals:

The stable group reported more pain between 10.00 and 14.00 and much the same pain as the neurotic group at other times of the day (Glynn and Lloyd, 1976, pp. 371-372).

The correlation between pain and alertness "was effectively zero" (p. 372).

Some researchers (e.g., Clark and Bindra, 1956) have reported a high positive correlation between pain threshold and pain tolerance. Others (Gelfand, Ullmann, and Krasner, 1963), however, found no significant correlation between these two measures. Gelfand (1964) attributed the inconsistent findings to differences in subject instructions and in the methods used to measure pain tolerance. A high positive correlation was found when permissive instructions were used ("This is not to see how much you can take.") and when pain tolerance was measured from the onset of stimulation. No significant correlations were found when nonpermissive instructions were given to the subjects. ("Keep your thumb down as long as possible.") and when pain tolerance was measured from the time of the subject's first report of pain (Gelfand, 1964, p. 37).

Gelfand compared pain thresholds and pain tolerance levels for two groups of subjects — one that received permissive instructions and one that received nonpermissive instructions. An ultrasonic unit was used to transmit sonic energy to the thumb of each subject. This procedure produces "a vigorous deep heating and painful reaction in organic tissue" (Gelfand, 1963, p. 406). Pain tolerance was measured as the duration of time in seconds from the subject's first report of pain (pain threshold) until he removed his thumb from the apparatus. Permissive instructions yielded a significantly lower pain tolerance than nonpermissive instructions. Pain threshold-pain tolerance correlations were negligible for both groups. Interestingly, Gelfand also calculated the pain threshold-pain tolerance correlations on the basis of Clark and Bindra's (1956) definition of pain tolerance which included pain threshold time. This technique yielded high positive correlations similar to those found by Clark and Bindra. These high correlations were explained by Gelfand (1964) as being:

> Statistical artifacts obtained by operationally defining pain tolerance time in such a way as to include pain threshold time. When these variables are defined as independent factors, a low nonsignificant correlation is found regardless of the instructions used (p. 41).

The relationship between birth order and pain tolerance was investigated by Schachter (in Gelfand, 1963). Gradually increasing intensities of electric shock were administered to female subjects who were instructed to indicate when the current was initially felt, when it became painful, and when it became unbearable. Schachter found that first-born and only children were "less willing or able to withstand the pain of maximum shock than . . . later children" (in Gelfand, 1963, p. 406). This finding was in part attributed to the greater anxiety and fear experienced by the first-born and only children in the face of an anxiety-producing situation. On the basis of these results and those of Beecher (in Gelfand, 1963) who observed that placebos were more effective in stressful situations, Gelfand (1963) hypothesized that first-born and only children should have a stronger placebo response than later-born children. Ultrasound stimulation was administered to two groups of female subjects in an investigation by Gelfand et al. (1963). One of the groups was also given a placebo which they thought was a pain-killing drug. They found that there was a tendency for first-born and only female children to show a greater increase in pain tolerance than later-born female children as a result of placebo medication. This difference, although observable, was not statistically significant.

SAFETY CONSIDERATIONS IN FARADIC AVERSION THERAPY

When a faradic stimulus is used in aversion therapy, safety should be a prime concern. The effect of electric shock on the body is determined by a number of factors. Three of these are voltage amplitude, the body's electrical resistance, and the amplitude of the current. A general rule concerning the interaction of these factors is that if body resistance remains constant, the higher the voltage, the higher the flow of current through the body. Total body resistance to electric shock consists of (a) the internal resistance of the body, and (b) the resistance of the skin at the contact points. The value of 1,000 Ω has been accepted by the National Fire Protection Association of the United States as the minimum body resistance value to be used when determining the maximum current output of a stimulus shocker (Butterfield, 1975).

The points at which electrodes are attached play an important role in the safety with which electric shock can be applied to the body. It would be unsafe, for example, to attach the electrodes at points "i" and "c" in Figure 27 because the current would flow through the chest area and could injure the heart. A current output as low as 80 μA may cause ventricular fibrillation (Butterfield, 1975). This is a condition whereby the ventricles of the

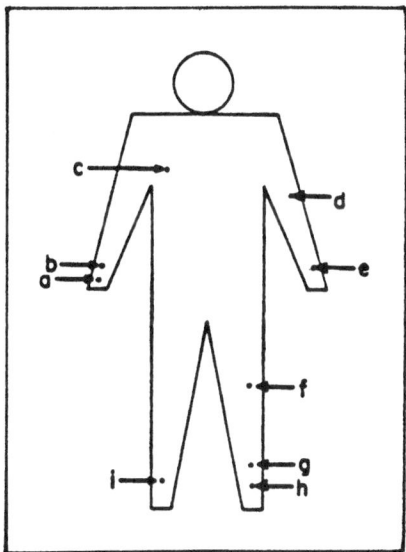

Figure 27. Safe and unsafe points of attachment of shock electrodes in man. From "Electric Shock — Safety Factors When Used for the Aversive Conditioning of Humans," by W. H. Butterfield, *Behavior Therapy*, 1975, *6*, 98-110.

heart contract ineffectively in a rapid, irregular, and uncoordin-
ated manner, thus disrupting cardiac output (*Blakiston's Gould
Medical Dictionary*, 1972). Safe attachments can be made to "the
same extremity with no other electrical connection being made any-
where on the body" (Butterfield, 1975, p. 100). The only safe
connection points would be "between d and e, between a and b,
and between any two of f, g, and h . . . . The most desirable
. . . would be between a and b or between g and h" (p. 100). In
this way, the current is localized.

A hazard exists when current output is allowed to flow (a) between an electrode and some other part of the apparatus, or (b)
between an electrode and a ground, such as a metal radiator.
Subject contact with either the equipment or the ground could
cause fatal injury (Butterfield, 1975).

Current that reverses its direction periodically (alternating
current) is less hazardous than current that flows in only one
direction (direct current). At least two reasons can be given for
this. First, direct current may cause chemical substances in either the electrode paste or the metal in the electrodes to penetrate
the skin and enter the body. Alternating current eliminates this
problem. Second, even low voltage direct current can produce
burns that are severe and slow to heal, especially if the electrodes
are attached too loosely or too tightly (Butterfield, 1975). Current density determines not only the level of current that must
flow to be sensed by the subject but also the heating effect of the
current. Current delivered through a small surface area such as
the point of a needle, for example, would have a greater density
and would be perceived as being more intense than the same current delivered through an electrode with a larger skin contact surface area. The smaller point of contact with the skin also increases the heating effect of the current and subsequently, the likelihood of burns.

The relationship between the intensity and duration of stimulus shock was discussed by Butterfield (1975):

> If the shock is longer than 0.1 sec "the current should be
> limited so that its ac rms or dc value is never greater than 15
> mA at 60 Hz. For shorter shocks, the energy content of the
> shock should be less than 0.2 W sec" (Bernstein, personal
> communication). In addition, current densities should be lim-
> ited to a maximum of 15 mA/cm^2 (p. 107).

In instances where commercially prepared faradic shockers are
unsuitable for specific research or treatment purposes, it may be
necessary for the researcher to construct his/her own stimulus

shocker. In such cases, it is extremely important that the apparatus be designed so that it can be safely used with human subjects. Applied researchers may find the six safety guidelines suggested to the author by Professor R. N. Scott (personal communication) of the Bio-Engineering Institute of the University of New Brunswick to be extremely useful. These include:

(a) the stimulator output should be isolated from ground, under all conditions of operation, leakage current less than 10 microamperes;

(b) the instrument leakage current with the ac line cord ungrounded should not exceed 10 microamperes;

(c) an emergency shutoff control, accessible to the subject at all times, should be provided in the experimental facility — perhaps a foot switch would be more suitable;

(d) all exposed metal parts of the experimental apparatus should be permanently grounded independent of the ac line cord, via a conductor not smaller than 16 AWG;

(e) no exposed metal should be situated within possible reach of the test subject — in particular, the use of push buttons with exposed metal bushings should be avoided;

(f) serious consideration should be given to the use of a low impedance ("constant voltage") stimulator rather than a high impedance ("constant current") stimulator, in order to eliminate the danger of skin burns due to poor electrode contact.

Considering the advantages of a faradic stimulus over other types of aversive stimuli and the safety with which an electrical stimulus can be administered, it seems that faradic aversion therapy is suitable for many types of behavioral problems.

3

Screening and Masking Techniques in Aversion Therapy

FACIAL SCREENING: INTRODUCTION

Facial screening is a recent technique that has been very effective in treating a variety of topographically different forms of maladaptive behaviors. The technique involves placing a facial screen, or bib, over the client's face contingent on the occurrence of the target behavior. The facial screen is usually made of a nonabrasive material such as terrycloth and must be large enough to cover the client's face. When applied, the bib is held loosely over the client's face for a stipulated duration (Lutzker, 1978; Singh, 1980; Zegiob, Jenkins, Becker, and Bristow, 1976).

Self-injurious behaviors have been the prime targets of facial screening. Lutzker (1978) found that a 20-year-old mentally retarded male's head- and face-slapping behavior was significantly reduced when facial screening was applied intermittently by his teachers. A terrycloth bib that measured 60 cm × 53 cm was held over the subject's face until the undesirable behavior had stopped for 3 seconds. Lutzker (1978) emphasized that the bib would not interfere with the client's breathing, even if it were held tightly over the face.

Singh, Beale, and Dawson (1981) treated self-injurious behavior in an 18-year-old, severely retarded girl who had an 11-year history of hitting herself about the face and lower jaw. At the time of treatment, she had been institutionalized for 13 years. Her social age on the Vineland Social Maturity Scale was equivalent to 2.2 years and her behavioral age on the Fairview Self-Help Scale was 16.9 months. Singh et al. (1981) contingently applied a 30 cm × 25 cm bib for durations of 3 seconds, 1 minute, and 3

minutes and found the 1-minute duration to be the most effective.
Compulsive hair-pulling was effectively treated by Barmann and
Vitali (1982) in three developmentally disabled persons. They
treated a nonverbal, 5-year-old Caucasian female with a mental
age of 16 months, a 9½-year-old Caucasian female with a mental
age of 18 months, and a 3-year-old Mexican-American male with
a low-severe to low-moderate range of retardation. The mean
training time was approximately 11 days and almost no regression
occurred during the 7-month follow-up period. Barmann and
Vitali used a 64 cm × 48 cm bib which they applied for 5 seconds
contingent on hair-pulling.

In Singh's (1980) study, facial screening rapidly suppressed
the self-injurious behavior of thumb-biting in an 11-month-old,
severely retarded boy. A terrycloth bib was used to cover the
infant's face for approximately 3 seconds immediately after thumb-
biting occurred. Twelve monthly follow-ups showed that improvement had been maintained.

Facial screening has been effective with a variety of other undesirable behaviors. For example, Barmann and Murray (1981)
successfully treated public genital self-stimulation in a 14-year-
old, severely retarded nonambulatory male in three different settings. A bib that was 64 cm long and 58 cm wide was applied for
5 seconds contingent on the occurrence of the self-stimulatory behavior. The mean training time was 5 days and the 6-month follow-up period indicated virtually no regression. Zegiob et al.
(1976) found that facial screening was very effective in suppressing disruptive hand-clapping in a 7-year-old nonverbal schizophrenic boy when the bib was applied for 10 seconds. If hand-
clapping occurred during the 10 seconds, the bib remained over
the boy's face until the behavior had stopped for 3 seconds.
Singh, Winton, and Dawson (1982) suppressed the screaming behavior of a 20-year-old profoundly retarded female whose social
age (Vineland Social Maturity Scale) was 1.4 years and whose behavioral age (Fairview Self-Help Scale) was 1.2 years. They reported that 1-minute periods of facial screening produced better
results than either 3-second or 30-second durations but did not
elaborate on this finding. The criterion for release from facial
screening was either a 1-minute, 3-second, or 30-second period
without screaming, depending on which condition was in effect.

As Lutzker and Wesch (in press) have indicated, a number
of techniques have been successful in reducing or eliminating self-
injurious behavior. It is difficult to predict, however, which
technique is more likely to be effective with a particular client.
In the case of facial screening, it has been observed that its ef-

fectiveness is usually obvious after the first few applications. Hence, the therapist is able to detect early in treatment whether or not facial screening is likely to be effective for the client. It has also been noted that the technique will likely be effective if a parent or staff member openly expresses the belief that the client will dislike the procedure. If the client hears spontaneous exclamations such as "he'll hate that," the technique of facial screening usually is very effective in suppressing the target behavior.

CRITICAL COMPONENTS OF FACIAL SCREENING

Few studies have determined the specific components of the technique that are responsible for its effectiveness. While application of facial screening in one phase of a study by Zegiob, Alford, and House (1978) produced dramatic results, their analysis of the separate phases of the technique failed to reveal which aspects were critical to its success. Neither placing the bib around the client's neck without facial screening nor holding the subject's head in the facial screening position contingent on self-hitting was effective in suppressing self-injurious behavior. On the basis of their results, Zegiob et al. concluded that visual blocking may be the critical component of the facial-screening technique.

Demetral and Lutzker (1980) studied several parameters of the facial-screening technique during their treatment of a 14-year-old male for hand-biting behavior and a 12-year-old female for chest-hitting behavior. Both preadolescents were severely mentally retarded. It was found that facial screening was most effective when it was response-contingent and when an opaque rather than a translucent bib was used. The latter finding seems to support the visual-blocking hypothesis of Zegiob and his colleagues. Researchers are now faced with the task of explaining *how* visual blocking contributes to the technique's effectiveness. One hypothesis might be that the technique is effective for young children because of the temporary period of darkness that is created when the bib is held over the client's face. Since children tend to be afraid of the dark, they may experience the application of the bib as fearful. This fear of the procedurally produced darkness would generally apply to younger children and one might expect that the impact of the darkness as an aversive stimulus would diminish with increasing age. The hypothesis that there would be greater response suppression with young children than with older children, however, has not been supported in the literature. The technique has been found to be very effective with 18- and 20-year-olds. The adolescents and adults in most studies, however, had very low mental and social ages, which may indicate that they possessed many of the fears characteristic of young children,[2] such as fear of the dark. If the visual-blocking component and possibly the procedurally produced darkness of facial screening are key features accounting for the technique's effectiveness, it seems that another effective procedure might be one in which the room is darkened whenever the target behavior occurs. This technique would have at least two advantages over facial screening. First, it would enable the therapist to *immediately* apply time-out contingent on the occurrence of the undesired behavior by activating a portable or remote-control light switch. In facial screening, immediate application may not always be possible if the therapist is not very close to the client when the target behavior occurs. A second advantage is that the technique would be extremely useful with clients who resist the facial screen or attempt to remove it once applied.

ADVANTAGES AND LIMITATIONS OF FACIAL SCREENING

Several advantages of the facial-screening technique are reported in the literature. First, the procedure involves the application of a nonpainful aversive stimulus in contrast to techniques that employ a painful stimulus such as faradic shock. Second, because there is little or no risk of injury to the client, this mildly aversive type of punishment is a socially acceptable procedure for controlling maladaptive behavior when other methods cannot be used because of ethical, legal, or pragmatic reasons (Barmann and Vitali, 1982; Lutzker, 1978; Singh et al., 1982; Zegiob et al., 1978). Third, maladaptive behavior is quickly suppressed, which is especially important when self-injury is the target behavior (Lutzker, 1978). Fourth, facial screening is an inexpensive procedure. Fifth, the procedure is uncomplicated and therefore can

---

[2]A study by Derevensky (1979) entitled "Children's Fears: A Developmental Comparison of Normal and Exceptional Children" suggested that exceptional children have a greater number and wider range of fears than normal children. In addition, most fears were found to be learned, realistic, and dependent on the child's intellectual and maturational level.

be easily learned and administered by individuals in the natural environment, given minimum training and supervision (Barmann and Murray, 1981; Barmann and Vitali, 1982; Lutzker, 1978). As Lutzker and Wesch (in press) have indicated, the treatment settings for facial screening have included the client's own home, institutions, group homes, and classrooms, and the procedure has been implemented by parents, nurses, graduate students, institutional staff, and bus aides. Sixth, teachers find the technique advantageous because it does not seriously disrupt classroom activities (Lutzker, 1978). Seventh, preliminary evidence indicates that the technique can be successfully applied intermittently (Lutzker, 1978, p. 512). This characteristic is important because teachers and parents may not always be able to apply the procedure contingent on every occurrence of the target behavior. There are two more advantages that relate to the parallel that has been drawn between facial screening and exclusion time-out (Apsche, Bacevich, Axelrod, and Keach, 1978; Singh, personal communication). First, if facial screening is a form of exclusion time-out, it has an advantage over seclusion time-out because the therapist does not have to move the client to a time-out room contingent on the occurrence of the target behavior. The other advantage relates more specifically to the contention of several researchers (Rincover, 1978; Rincover, Cook, Peoples, and Packard, 1979; Rincover and Koegel, 1977; Rincover, Newsom, Lovaas, and Koegel, 1977) that many self-stimulatory and self-injurious behaviors are maintained by their sensory consequences. In seclusion time-out, there is ample opportunity for the client to engage in these self-reinforcing behaviors while he is alone in the time-out room. In facial screening, however, the client remains in his natural setting where he can be seen by the therapist. This reduces the likelihood that the individual will engage in the target behavior without it being met by appropriate remedial action by the therapist.

The chief disadvantage of facial screening is that it requires a one-to-one therapist/client ratio (Singh et al., 1982). A second limitation, which is unique to the technique itself, is that uncooperative clients may remove the facial screen as soon as it is applied. Temporary resistance to facial screening, however, usually disappears within the first few sessions (Singh, 1980; Singh et al., 1981: Singh et al., 1982; Zegiob et al., 1976). A third potential limitation is that there is opportunity for interpersonal friction between the therapist and client because they are not separated from each other as they are, for example, in seclusion time-out.

SELF-APPLICATION OF FACIAL SCREENING

Facial screening usually involves direct therapist intervention but self-application of the technique has been observed to occur in several studies. The 2½-year-old developmentally normal girl in the Singh et al. (1982) study was observed self-administering the facial screen consequent to her screaming behavior if her mother delayed in applying the procedure. The 7-year-old schizophrenic boy in the Zegiob et al. (1976) study occasionally pulled the bib over his face when he engaged in inappropriate hand-clapping. It is possible that children might be taught or cued with a "bug-in-the-ear" device[3] (Stumphauzer, 1971) to use the facial-screening bib themselves after each occurrence of the target behavior.

VISUAL SCREENING

McGonigle, Duncan, Cordisco, and Barrett (1982) investigated the effectiveness of a procedure called visual screening on stereotypic and self-injurious behaviors of four developmentally disabled children. This procedure is similar to facial screening but does not require special equipment such as a bib. The therapist places one hand over the client's eyes while holding the back of the client's head with the other hand. Duration of each visual-screening application in the McGonigle et al. (1982) study was a minimum of 5 seconds, with the criterion for release from visual screening being that nondisruptive behavior occurred following expiration of the minimum time requirement. The results indicated that "the visual screening treatment procedure was effective in significantly reducing the frequency of stereotypic responding for each child" (p. 464). Follow-up data were collected at intervals

---

[3]A "bug-in-the-ear" device enables the therapist to directly communicate with a trainee without disrupting an ongoing activity. There are two major uses of the apparatus. First, it enables the clinician to unobtrusively prompt the trainee (e.g., "Apply the facial screen now") and second, it enables the therapist to provide immediate social reinforcement to the trainee (e.g., "That's good!"). The device can be constructed for under $5.00. Other than a tape recorder and a microphone with an on-off switch, all that is needed is an earphone, extension cord, and a miniature microphone (Stumphauzer, 1971).

ranging from 2 to 18 months and in each case, "no observed instances of the targeted responses were reported" (p. 464).
McGonigle et al. (1982) concluded that visual screening is a quick
and easily administered procedure that is effective with a variety
of stereotypic and self-stimulatory behaviors. It can be implemented with minimal training and without special equipment in both
a classroom and group-home setting. Results are similar to those
found in studies using facial screening.

Another variation of visual screening was used by Apsche et
al. (1978) to reduce aggressive behaviors in a 17-year-old mildly
retarded institutionalized girl. Their procedure involved the use
of an eyescreen or blindfold which was 2 inches wide and made of
an opaque cloth held together by a piece of elastic. The girl was
restrained and the eyescreen placed around her head for a 10-
minute time-out period after every occurrence of the inappropriate behavior. When this procedure was compared with a contingent observation time-out procedure, it was found that during the
restraint/eyescreen phase of the study, all target behaviors were
reduced markedly and immediately, whereas during restraint/con-
tingent observation, disruptive behaviors either continued at the
baseline level or increased in frequency. According to Apsche et
al. (1978), the eyescreen procedure has an advantage over facial
screening in that once the screen is applied, it does not have to
be held in place. This procedure would seem to be easier for a
single individual to implement with clients who are resistant. Another advantage is that there need not be any concern for the
screen interfering with the client's breathing. Although a facial
screen supposedly does not hinder breathing, the use of an eyescreen eliminates the possibility of such an occurrence.

THEORETICAL EXPLANATIONS OF FACIAL SCREENING

According to Achenbach (1974, p. 362), four chief models of
aversive control of behavior have been conceptualized within the
framework of respondent and operant conditioning paradigms.
These are:

1. Removal of positive reinforcement following a response to
    be eliminated [negative punishment].
2. Application of aversive stimuli following a response to be
    eliminated [positive punishment].
3. Removal of aversive stimuli to reinforce an escape or
    avoidance response [negative reinforcement].

4. Making neutral or positive stimuli aversive by pairing
    them with events that are already aversive [classical aver-
    sive conditioning].

Several of these models have been used to explain the effectiveness of facial screening. Alford (personal communication) indicates that "some debate continues about whether it [facial
screening] removes reinforcement [Model 1--negative punishment]
or is an aversive stimulus event: punisher [Model 2--positive
punishment]." The most common explanation is that it is response-contingent punishment; that is, a procedure in which a
mildly aversive stimulus is presented[4] each time the target behavior occurs (Barmann and Murray, 1981; Barmann and Vitali, 1982;
Lutzker, 1978; Singh, 1980; Zegiob et al., 1976; Zegiob et al.,
1978). Alford (personal communication) favors the positive-punishment model and conceptualizes facial screening as:

> A non-painful punisher which might be useful in decelerating
> high frequency abnormal or disruptive behavior thereby pro-
> viding or allowing more opportunity for appropriate adaptive
> behaviors to be emitted and reinforced.

Zegiob (personal communication) describes facial screening as a
"fairly effective, efficient punisher" and is another proponent of
the positive-punishment model. He concluded that:

> Facial screening has been classified in the research and treat-
> ment literature as a punishment procedure; while only mildly
> aversive, facial screening does cause a decrease in the rate/
> frequency of the target behavior. Thus, it fits the accepted
> definition of a punishment stimulus.

------

[4]The term "aversive event" is not a synonym for unpleasant stimulus. An event is aversive if it occurs after the response and
the response then decreases in frequency. Defining punishment
in terms of its *function*, or the effect it has on the rate of occurrence of behavior, is useful because it helps to clarify that the
type of event presented, that is, the pleasantness or unpleasantness of the stimulus, has nothing to do with the technical definition of punishment. A functional definition of punishment indicates that a positive event, such as praise, would be defined
as an aversive stimulus — a "punisher" — if the behavior were
reduced after the positive event was presented (Deitz and Hummel, 1978, pp. 77-80).

Singh (personal communication) notes the close resemblance between facial screening and exclusion time-out. In exclusion time-out, the individual is removed from the activity and deprived of social interaction. He is allowed to remain in the room but is unable to observe the behavior of his peers (Apsche et al., 1978). Similarly, in facial screening, the placing of the bib over the client's face renders him unable to observe his peers and although he is allowed to remain in the room, his social interaction is limited.

The essential feature of a time-out from positive reinforcement procedure, according to Leitenberg (1965a), is a period of time during which positive reinforcement is no longer available. Applying the bib in facial screening removes positive reinforcement and hence appears to qualify the technique as a form of time-out. While facial screening resembles exclusion time-out, it appears to be very different from contingent observation and seclusion time-out. [5]

Achenbach (1974) has used three models of aversive control of behavior to explain the operation of time-out procedures:

> According to Model 1, the effect of time-out is to cut off all possibilities for positive reinforcement. Thus, any positive reinforcements previously supporting the behavior are removed and the behavior should extinguish. However, the effects of time-out are also interpretable under Model 2, the contingent application of aversive stimuli (punishment), because being closed in a room and losing positive reinforcers are both aversive. According to Model 3, time-out may result in the conditioning of nondisruptive responses to whatever stimuli previously elicited disruptive responses because the new responses are reinforced by avoidance of isolation or escape from it if termination of time-out is contingent on cessation of disruptive behavior (p. 363).

---

[5] In contingent observation, the offending individual is removed to the periphery of the activity, deprived of reinforcing materials, and is instructed to observe the activities of compliant peers. Later the offending individual is allowed to rejoin the activity . . . . In seclusion time-out, the offending individual is physically removed from the activity room and is placed in an isolation area, which precludes social interaction and other reinforcing events (Apsche et al., 1978, p. 2).

ISSUES AND GUIDELINES IN THE USE OF SCREENING

Since screening and masking techniques in aversion therapy share many characteristics with time-out procedures, it is important to address several issues that are critical to the effective operation of time-out. These are (a) the optimal duration of time-out, (b) the effect of increasing or decreasing time-out durations during treatment, and (c) the criteria for the client's release from time-out. In a review of several studies, White, Nielsen, and Johnson (1972) found that time-out durations varied from 3 seconds to 2 hours, although many researchers used durations of less than 15 minutes. In their own study, White et al. found that seclusion time-out durations of 15 and 30 minutes decreased the deviant behavior equally as well. The greatest effect was observed when a short duration of 1 minute preceded the use of longer durations. When the 1-minute time-out followed the application of longer durations, it was not as effective in suppressing behavior as when it preceded them. Because of this sequence effect, White et al. reported that it is preferable to begin with brief time-out durations. If these are ineffective, the option is available to increase the durations. Johnston (1972) has recommended the use of brief time-out intervals for two reasons:

> All responses occurring during the time-out are unavoidably paired with the aversive stimuli in the situation. Thus, the longer the time-out period, the greater the probability of pairing desirable responses with aversive stimuli. Longer time-out periods also serve to remove the subject from treatment sessions for greater periods of time, thus lessening the opportunity for reinforcement of appropriate behaviors (pp. 1039-1040).

White et al. (1972, p. 1039) have indicated that release from time-out should occur when the punished response terminates, at the end of a predetermined time after the punished behavior has ceased, or following the occurrence of some appropriate response. The second criterion appears to be the one that most researchers of the effects of facial screening have employed (Lutzker, 1978; Lutzker and Spencer, 1974; Singh et al., 1982; Zegiob et al., 1976).

It is recognized that empirical data from clinical studies will be required to determine if time-out guidelines apply to screening and masking techniques in aversion therapy. It seems reasonable to expect, however, that duration guidelines would be similar for both time-out procedures and facial screening. Long durations of facial screening may have the same disadvantages that Johnston (1972) has indicated for time-out. While he recommended brief durations, it is conceivable that there would be potential problems in facial screening with durations that are too brief. If a facial screen is applied for only a few seconds, it is possible that the undesirable behavior may still be occurring after the screen is removed. If the target behavior continues to occur, it is doing so without resulting in punishment, and may even be associated with positive reinforcement. This would reduce the efficacy of the facial-screening technique. The procedure of continuing to apply the screen until the target behavior has stopped appears to eliminate this problem.

SENSORY EXTINCTION: INTRODUCTION

It is often difficult in applied settings to identify the reinforcer of a particular undesirable behavior. Removing as many potentially reinforcing stimuli as possible when implementing time-out may be effective in suppressing the target behavior, but it is not always successful (Johnston, 1972). According to Rincover (1978), some behaviors, such as self-stimulation, are maintained by their sensory consequences rather than by social or environmental stimuli. For this type of behavior, a punishment procedure that removes all social reinforcement is not likely to be effective. Putting the client in a time-out room, for example, merely provides him with the opportunity to further engage in self-stimulatory behavior and to experience the sensory reinforcement that has been responsible for maintaining the behavior (Gelfand and Hartmann, 1975, p. 180). Rincover et al. (1977) referred to sensory reinforcement as "the unconditioned property of sensory events to increase the probability of behaviors they follow" (p. 313). When it is suspected that an undesirable behavior such as hand-flapping is being maintained by sensory stimulation, consideration should be given to treating the behavior by sensory extinction. Rincover (1978) described sensory extinction as a new procedure "in which certain sensory consequences are masked or removed in an attempt to assess whether self-stimulation is operant behavior maintained by sensory reinforcement" (p. 301).

By manipulating the sensory consequences of self-stimulatory behaviors in three autistic children, Rincover (1978) found that finger-flapping and object-spinning were reliably decreased when a particular sensory consequence was removed or masked and that the behaviors increased when that consequence was permitted.

Removing the auditory feedback from plate-spinning behavior by carpeting the tabletop was effective in significantly reducing the behavior. After returning to the baseline condition and implementing a procedure by which only the visual feedback of the plate-spinning behavior was removed by using a blindfold, the behavior remained at a relatively high rate. When auditory feedback was again removed, and visual feedback permitted, the behavior was extinguished and was maintained "at or near 0 over a period of 2 months" (p. 306). These findings suggest that plate-spinning behavior had been "maintained by its auditory consequences and could be extinguished by removing those auditory consequences" (p. 306). For another child, Rincover (1978) masked the proprioceptive feedback from finger-flapping by using a small vibratory mechanism that was taped to the back of the child's hand. The device, which did not restrict hand movements, generated a low-intensity, high-frequency pulsation which approximated the proprioceptive stimulation received from finger-flapping. This procedure reduced the behavior to a very low rate and retained its effectiveness over several weeks. As with plate-spinning, removing the visual consequences of the finger-flapping behavior did not significantly reduce its frequency.

In a more recent study, Williamson, Coon, Lemoine, and Cohen (1983) found that sensory extinction significantly reduced the inappropriate behavior of toy-throwing and that withdrawing the procedure resulted in a substantial increase in the behavior. Williamson et al.'s procedure of attaching a child's toy to a 12-inch string that was tied to his wrist enabled him to perform the throwing movements but removed the natural visual consequences of "observing the objects fly across the room" (p. 206). Toy-throwing behavior was successfully reduced by this procedure which Williamson et al. interpreted as support for Rincover's sensory reinforcement hypothesis. They emphasized that sensory extinction does not prevent the occurrence of an inappropriate behavior but rather eliminates or masks the natural sensory consequences of the behavior. Prior to the work of Rincover and his colleagues (Rincover, 1978; Rincover and Koegel, 1977; Rincover et al., 1977; Rincover et al., 1979) and more recent studies (Williamson et al., 1983) on the role of sensory reinforcement in motivating self-stimulatory behaviors, extinction procedures[6] had been used

----

[6]Extinction refers to the cessation of reinforcement of a response which leads to a reduction or elimination of the response

primarily to suppress behaviors maintained by social reinforcement. The efficacy of extinction has now been extended to the treatment of behaviors for which reinforcement is purely sensory.

Interestingly, Barmann and Vitali (1982) have cited sensory extinction as a possible explanation for the effectiveness of their facial-screening procedure in eliminating compulsive hair-pulling behavior. They stated that "since the children in this study liked to both look at and play with their hair after pulling it, then the facial screening procedure may have acted as a vehicle for removing the visual sensory reinforcement, thereby extinguishing the hair-pulling behavior" (p. 741). This statement seems to align with Rincover's rationale for his sensory extinction procedure of using a blindfold to remove the visual sensory consequences of self-stimulatory behaviors exhibited by three autistic children. Another point in favor of a sensory extinction explanation for Barmann and Vitali's results is that a graphic illustration of their data appeared to "represent that of an extinction curve, as opposed to the abrupt changes typically achieved with a punishment procedure" (p. 741). It appears that such an explanation for the effectiveness of facial screening may be a viable one, especially for behaviors that are maintained by visual sensory stimulation.

ADVANTAGES OF SENSORY EXTINCTION

The literature has indicated that there is a consensus among the researchers of sensory extinction that this procedure has several positive features and advantages over other methods of behavioral control. The first and foremost is that it has been found

---

(Kazdin, 1980, p. 38). It is the process of "disconnecting" the relationship between a response and its consequences (Craighead, Kazdin, and Mahoney, 1981). Kazdin (1980) provided a cogent distinction between extinction and punishment when he commented that "in extinction, no consequence follows the response; that is, an event is not taken away nor is one presented. In punishment, some aversive event follows a response or some positive event is taken away" (p. 38). In everyday life, the usual use of extinction is in the form of ignoring behavior; for example, a mother may ignore her child's whining or a teacher may ignore those children who talk out in class without raising their hands. In both examples, the reinforcer (attention, approval, or sympathy) is no longer available (Kazdin, 1980).

to be a very effective treatment for self-stimulation, producing
dramatic reduction in the rate of the target behavior (Devany and
Rincover, 1982; Rincover, 1978; Rincover et al., 1979). Self-
stimulatory behaviors pose a serious challenge to treatment and
have been found to be resistant to social extinction and other procedures such as time-out. Second, the procedure of sensory extinction is relatively efficient, requiring minimal staff training and
child supervision, and only a small investment of time and money
(Devany and Rincover, 1982). These features make it suitable for
use in the classroom or in institutions, where it is often difficult
to provide a one-to-one client/therapist ratio. Third, no serious
ethical concerns have been raised by nonprofessionals such as
parents, classroom peers, or staff who have served as therapeutic
agents. Unlike many other methods of behavioral control, sensory
extinction reduces inappropriate behavior without the use of aversive contingencies. Fourth, the results have been shown to be
maintained over time without the use of other interventions (Williamson et al., 1983).

LIMITATIONS OF SENSORY EXTINCTION

Several limitations of extinction procedures have been mentioned in the literature. First, the therapist may encounter difficulty in identifying the reinforcer of an undesirable behavior.
Since the efficacy of a sensory-extinction procedure is contingent
on identifying and removing the reinforcer, failure to do so would
render the procedure ineffective. An illustration of a mistakenly
identified reinforcer would be removing or masking the auditory
feedback associated with object-throwing when the actual reinforcer is the visual feedback received when the object is thrown
across the room. As Rincover et al. (1979) suggested, some behaviors may have multiple sensory reinforcers which may necessi-
tate the use of elaborate extinction procedures in order to identify
the actual reinforcers. A second problem that may be encountered
when attempting to use an extinction procedure is controlling or
removing the reinforcer once it has been identified. If the reinforcing consequence cannot be eliminated, as is sometimes the case
with proprioceptive consequences (Devany and Rincover, 1982),
extinction cannot be effectively implemented because, by definition, extinction means withholding reinforcement (Deitz and Hummel, 1978). Third, an extinction procedure may cause an initial
increase in the frequency of the target behavior (Deitz and Hummel, 1978). If such a phenomenon is intolerable, as in the case

of self-injurious behavior, extinction would not be an appropriate procedure to use. Fourth, a behavior often reappears after it has been eliminated by extinction. This problem of spontaneous recovery is not usually serious but it is crucial that the misbehavior not be reinforced when it reappears; otherwise, it may be reestablished at the same or even greater frequency than before treatment (Deitz and Hummel, 1978, pp. 149-150). Fifth, some negative emotional side-effects such as rage, crying, withdrawal, frustration, and aggression may be evident upon using extinction procedures (Deitz and Hummel, 1978). The extent to which these responses occur should be monitored and considered when deciding whether or not an extinction procedure is appropriate.

REINFORCING FUNCTION OF SELF-STIMULATION

Sensory extinction has been found to be very effective in reducing or eliminating self-stimulatory behaviors such as rhythmical rocking, hand- and arm-flapping, and object-twirling. These behaviors interfere with learning and may also be ostracizing if people are frightened or repelled by them. It may not be desirable, however, to eliminate self-stimulation completely. Since self-stimulatory behaviors can be powerfully reinforcing, it may be beneficial to harness this function and use self-stimulation to reinforce appropriate behavior (Devany and Rincover, 1982). Their assumption was that, if low-rate behaviors such as appropriate play or social behaviors are associated with an opportunity to engage in an identified high-rate, self-stimulatory behavior, the appropriate behaviors should increase in frequency.

Sensory-extinction procedures are sometimes designed and implemented for the purpose of identifying the sensory reinforcers that maintain self-stimulatory behavior. By systematically removing the auditory, visual, or proprioceptive sensory consequences of self-stimulation, a child's most preferred sensory reinforcer can be identified (Devany and Rincover, 1982). Activities and objects can then be provided to the child to produce this particular sensory consequence when engaging in appropriate behavior. Reduction of excessive and disruptive self-stimulation by sensory extinction and concomitant positive gains in appropriate play behavior were found by Devany and Rincover (1982) to be "durable over a period of months without external reinforcers for play or restraints on self-stimulation" (p. 132). Rincover et al. (1977) found that three types of sensory stimulation, that is, a strobe light, music, and oscillating windshield wipers, produced very high rates of responding on a bar-pressing task by four autistic children. Each child's preferred type of sensory stimulation was provided for 5 seconds contingent on performing five bar presses. The high rate of responding remained durable over the 52 sessions, which demonstrates that self-stimulatory reinforcers are very resistant to satiation. Rincover et al. (1977) found that, although the children eventually satiated on their preferred sensory event, a small change in the topography of that event, e.g., a new speed of wiper movement or a change in frequency of the strobe light, functioned to recover the high rate of responding and maintained this rate over time.

Rincover and Devany (1978) allowed the three children in their study to play for 5 to 10 seconds with objects such as keys, twigs, and bubbles after each correct response on a task such as sentence completion or letter discrimination. In contrast to the frequent breaks that are required when food is used as a reinforcer, the children sometimes worked for 300 trials or more before satiation occurred. When children's responses to food and self-stimulatory reinforcers were compared (Rincover and Devany, 1979), it was found that they worked longer and learned more when the self-stimulatory reinforcers were used. This illustrates that sensory reinforcers are very powerful and more resistant to satiation than edible reinforcers.

Concern has been expressed by parents and professionals that using self-stimulation as a reinforcer may lead to an increase in the rate of self-stimulation outside treatment and that it may strengthen self-stimulatory behavior and make it more resistant to later treatment (Devany and Rincover, 1982). Rincover and Devany (1979) found, however, that there was no change in the rate of self-stimulation outside treatment when self-stimulation was used as a reinforcer during treatment. They also found that extinction procedures were effective in rapidly decreasing self-stimulation, even if self-stimulatory activities had been used over a long period of time as reinforcers. Devany and Rincover (1982) concluded that "the procedure of harnessing self-stimulation as a reinforcer could prove to be a valuable tool for the *elimination* of self-stimulation" (p. 138).

4
Theories of Aversive Control of Behavior

CLASSICAL CONDITIONING

One of several theoretical formulations discussed by Hallam and Rachman (1972) to account for the effectiveness of aversion therapy was classical conditioning. This model predicts that approach responses to a deviant stimulus will be replaced by aversive responses after therapy. The following is a specific illustration of this theoretical proposition:

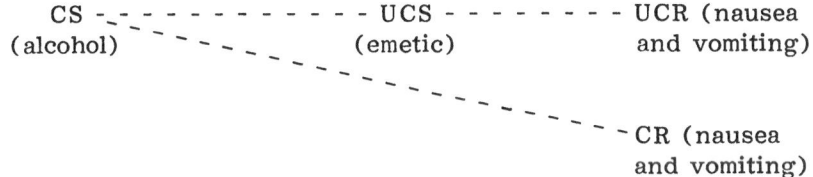

CS - - - - - - - - - - - - - - UCS - - - - - - - - - UCR (nausea
(alcohol)   (emetic)   and vomiting)

- - - CR (nausea
and vomiting)

Rachman and Teasdale (1969) have reported, however, that the conditioned response to the deviant stimulus is usually indifference and not aversion. A similar view was expressed by Lovibond (1970) who stated that "the punished behavior is not merely held in abeyance, but the motivation to perform the act is reduced" (p. 89). McConaghy (1972) reported that observations from his chemical aversion treatment studies of homosexual behavior directly contradicted the Pavlovian prediction of UCR-CR similarity. The subjects were given apomorphine, which induced nausea subsequent to their viewing pictures of nude men. McConaghy indicated that the CR of nausea was *not* experienced after therapy upon subsequent exposure to similar pictures. In other words, the conditioned response expected as a result of aversion therapy was not observed. In 1971, McConaghy employed a backward conditioning technique with a faradic stimulus to treat homosexual behavior. The effect of this backward conditioning procedure in which subjects "received a series of shocks, following each of which they viewed the slide of a male" (McConaghy, 1971, p. 1224) were compared to the effects of a standard forward classical conditioning procedure. McConaghy reported that backward conditioning produced about the same results as forward conditioning.

Chemical, rather than faradic aversion therapy, more closely approximates classical conditioning because the CR that is produced is similar to the UCR (Hallam, Rachman, and Falkowski, 1972). When shock is used as an aversive stimulus, it is difficult to determine what CR, if any, is produced and what the individual experiences outside therapy when he encounters the deviant stimulus. The shock produces a pain UCR during conditioning trials but the individual would be unlikely to experience pain when presented with the negatively conditioned stimulus during test trials or during natural posttreatment occurrences of the stimulus. Instead, it seems that he would probably report anxiety, which Mowrer described as a "conditioned pain response" (cited in Hallam et al., 1972, p. 1). Hallam et al. asserted that a strictly Pavlovian interpretation predicts that changes in GSR and cardiac functioning should accompany conditioned anxiety. In this respect, they stated:

1. Plainly, if UCS (shock) → pain/anxiety plus GSR/cardiac changes
2. then, CS (deviant stimulus) → UCS (Xn)
3. should lead to CS (deviant stimulus) → pain/anxiety plus GSR/cardiac change (Hallam et al., 1972, p. 2).

These researchers studied the subjective experiences of individuals who had previously undergone faradic aversion therapy. Information was collected from six middle-class alcoholics, five lower-class alcoholics, and five sexual deviates. None of the subjects studied by Hallam et al. reported experiencing fear or anxiety when in the presence of the deviant stimulus after treatment. The major changes in feelings toward the deviant stimuli were the acquisition of repulsion or indifference to a particular deviant stimulus and "not fear or anxiety" (Hallam et al., 1972, p. 4). Four of the middle-class alcoholics reported that they had experienced an unpleasant change in the smell and taste of alcohol. All four, three of whom said they were now repulsed by the smell and taste, were successes. This appeared to be the only group that developed a true aversion, but as Hallam et al. noted, "the type of treatment administered to these patients included sessions during which they were required to smell and taste a selection of alcoholic drinks" (p. 3). The other alcoholics were not required to taste alcohol during treatment nor were they permitted to consume it between treatment sessions. It is interesting to note that the taste aversion that developed with the middle-class alcoholics could not have been predicted from classical conditioning with faradic shock. Taste aversion would be predicted, however, if an emetic rather than a faradic stimulus had been used as the UCS. Following Hallam et al.'s argument, it is clear that the CR of taste or smell aversion to the alcoholic stimuli is very different indeed from the UCR of pain/anxiety experienced during training trials in which the alcoholic stimuli were paired with stimulus shock.

It is reasonable to expect that because a faradic stimulus was used, subjects would experience anxiety or tension during the treatment period. Only one of the subjects, however, reported feeling tension on the night before a treatment session. Even more surprising was the finding that only four subjects reported being tense as near as a half hour before a treatment session. Several subjects reported tension during treatment.

In a second part of the same study, Hallam et al. investigated whether or not autonomic responses to deviant stimuli used in treatment "will change in the direction of increased responsivity" (p. 5). An aversion therapy group and a control group, both comprised of chronic alcoholics, were compared for changes in physiological responses to alcoholic and nonalcoholic stimuli. Aversion therapy subjects were shocked under two conditions: (a) in association with fantasies about their drinking behavior which were stimulated by slides depicting pubs or bottles of alcohol; (b) while looking at, smelling, or tasting their favorite alcoholic drinks. Subjects in both the aversion therapy and control groups received in-patient hospital care which included group therapy and medication. Hence, the control group was called a "control-treatment" group.

Hallam et al. (1972) were unable to find significant differences between groups in heart rate and galvanic skin response to alcoholic stimuli after treatment. Nonetheless, a significant difference was found in heart rate responsivity between successes and failures, irrespective of whether they were aversion therapy or control subjects. Reviewing the data just cited, Hallam et al. concluded that:

> *Success* may be attributable to the common therapeutic vari-
> ables — namely, hospital in-patient care combined with group
> meetings [and] non-interpretative weekly sessions of psycho-
> therapy (p.13).

In view of the findings discussed, it seems that a Pavlovian interpretation of aversion therapy has limited explanatory value.

CHANGE IN VALENCE OR FUNCTION OF DEVIANT STIMULUS

Marks and Sartorius (in Hallam and Rachman, 1972) have noted that "the patients' most common report after aversion therapy is that the deviant stimulus has lost its attraction and interest for them" (p. 345). This change in the valence of the deviant stimulus is the basis for a second theoretical explanation of the effectiveness of aversion therapy. Evidence seems to indicate that "patients perceive differences in the qualities of the deviant stimulus even though there has been no physical change in stimulus attributes" (Hallam and Rachman, 1972, pp. 345-346).

ATTITUDE CHANGE

A third theoretical proposition suggests that "changes of attitude can mediate behavioural changes" (Hallam and Rachman, 1972, p. 347). Marks, Gelder, and Bancroft (1970), for example, found that attitude changes occurred in sexual deviates during aversion therapy. The following excerpt from the Marks et al. (1970) research describes their attitude measurement procedure:

> *Attitudes*: Patients' attitudes were measured on 10 semantic differential scales. On the basis of principal component analyses the ten scales were grouped into three factors — *general evaluation* (3 scales: pleasant-unpleasant, good-bad, kind-cruel), *sexual evaluation* (4 scales: seductive-repulsive, sexy-sexless, exciting-dull, erotic-frigid) and *anxiety* (3 scales: placid-jittery, calm-anxious, relaxed-tense). The patient rated twenty concepts on each of the 10 scales: 4 concepts judged to be most relevant to his particular sexual deviation (e.g., *woman's dress, high heeled shoes*); 3 concepts concerning normal sexual relations (*my wife/fiancée/ girlfriend, sexual intercourse*); 9 concerning matters relevant to his clinical state and treatment (*my G.P., psychiatrists, the Maudsley Hospital, my father, my mother, myself, myself as I would like to be, people with the same trouble as me, and electric shocks*) and 4 control concepts (pp. 174-175).

Changes in the subjects' attitudes toward the four sexually deviant concepts at the end of aversion therapy correlated positively and significantly with their improvement rating at the end of treatment and with the decrease in the number of deviant acts reported during posttreatment follow-up.

In their 1972 investigation, Hallam et al. tested the hypothesis that after faradic aversion therapy for alcoholism, "an attitude-change signifying aversion to the deviant activity will develop" (p. 5). The subjects' attitudes toward drinking and neutral slides were measured before and after treatment by means of a 7-point scale. This scale measured the factors of:

'General evaluation' (good-bad, kind-cruel, attractive-unat-tractive), 'taste' (appetizing-repulsive, tasty-distasteful, pleasant-unpleasant), 'anxiety' (makes-me-calm-makes-me-anxious, alarming-relaxing) and 'danger' (harmless-harmful, dangerous-safe). Ratings were averaged for each factor over the five 'drinking' and five 'neutral' slides (Hallam et al., 1972, p. 7).

Prior to the experiment, aversion therapy and control subjects rated the drinking slides as "slightly good, tasty, harmless and relaxing" (Hallam et al., 1972, p. 9), while at posttreatment, all subjects rated the drinking slides as slightly bad, distasteful, anxiety-provoking, and dangerous. One attitude difference between the two groups was that after treatment, both neutral and drinking slides were reported as being more distasteful to the aversion therapy group than to the control group. Irrespective of groups, no difference was observed between the successes and failures on the taste factor. Hence, Hallam et al. concluded that there was "no direct relationship between the distaste, which developed in the aversion therapy group, and clinical outcome" (p. 11). Slight increases in posttreatment anxiety to the alcoholic stimuli were reflected in the anxiety ratings of the aversion therapy and control-treatment groups. The between-groups difference, however, was not significant.

Hallam and Rachman (1972) pointed out a possible limitation of self-rating measures for assessing attitude change, as reflected in their statement:

Patients are normally strongly dissuaded from pursuing their deviant habits while treatment is in progress and so behavioural indices are confounded by instruction effects and cannot be readily correlated with attitudinal change (p. 347).

These researchers noted that attitudes about a deviant stimulus constitute more than a positive or negative evaluation of the stimulus. They considered it desirable, therefore, to obtain information about an individual's "cognitive appraisal of his deviant behaviour" (p. 347) to assist in the planning of treatment. In this respect, Hallam and Rachman asserted that:

> Only those patients who perceive some dissonance between their deviant behavior and their self-image are likely to refer themselves or to be selected for treatment (pp. 347-348).

COGNITIVE DISSONANCE

A fourth argument for the effectiveness of aversion therapy is inherent in the theory of cognitive dissonance. A study by Carlin and Armstrong (1968) provides evidence for the importance of cognitive variables in aversion therapy. In reporting their experimental procedure, Carlin and Armstrong indicated that:

> For each S electrodes were attached to the third finger and wrist of his nonpreferred hand. Current was adjusted slowly upward to a point that S identified as extremely unpleasant, but tolerable.
>
> The conditioning group was instructed to light a cigarette and to puff on command. They were signaled to puff every 25 seconds and were shocked on a 75% variable interval schedule with a shock stimulus of 5-second duration. After 12 puffs S extinguished the cigarette, rested 5 minutes, the shock was readjusted, and then S smoked a second cigarette. The procedure described above was repeated for this cigarette. Each day for 4 consecutive days the C group Ss filled out reports of smoking level, electrodes were attached, shock adjusted upwards, and the two cigarettes smoked. They received 18 pairings of shock with inhalation of cigarette smoke over a series of 24 puffs.
>
> A "pseudoconditioning" condition was devised in which there was a degree of apparent relevance to the treatment of smoking and in which there were the cognitive elements of a conditioning paradigm but also in which S engaged in no smoking behavior. The Ss viewed 27 slides for 15 seconds each. Nine of these slides were smoking relevant. The S received electric shock during the last 5 seconds exposure of nine randomly selected slides. After the entire sequence of 27 slides, S rested 5 minutes, the shock was readjusted, and again he

viewed the series receiving shock of 5-second duration in connection with nine randomly selected slides. An average of
3.12 smoking relevant slides were paired with the shock on
each series. As with the conditioning group this procedure
was carried out on each of 4 consecutive days. This arrange-
ment was employed as the "pseudoconditioning" situation
rather than the pairing of random shock with actual smoking
behavior, since the latter might not result in pseudoconditioning at all. Rather, it could result in the pairing of aversive
stimulation to some segment of the smoking behavior sequence.
Thus, aversive stimuli were applied, but contiguous with no
smoking behavior.
The Ss in the Con [Control] group received the same adjust-
ment of shock level as was described for the other two groups.
After maximal shock level was determined, each S was told
that he was going to receive subliminal shock and without his
knowledge the shock apparatus was turned off. Except for
his receiving no shock whatsoever, the Con S was subjected
to the same procedure as was the C S (pp. 675-676).

Smoking was significantly reduced in all three groups which suggested that behavior change was not a function of conditioning.
Carlin and Armstrong (1968, p. 674) attributed the behavior
change to factors such as "belief, expectancy, and cognitive con-
sistency." They further explained that an individual who commits
himself to faradic aversion therapy experiences cognitive dissonance. In other words, it would be difficult for a subject to continue to smoke and at the same time maintain the belief that he had
made a "wise commitment of his time and effort through a process
involving considerable physical pain" (p. 675).

Tedeschi, Schlenker, and Bonoma have proposed that cognitive dissonance theory has several limitations. Their criticisms
were outlined by Hallam and Rachman (1972):

(a) People seem able to tolerate a great deal of inconsistency
in their behaviour and beliefs, (b) people do not usually avoid
tension-arousing information, (c) it is not always possible to
make clear predictions from the theory, (d) many studies
have not been replicated and (e) the origin of the motivational state aroused by inconsistency has not been explained (p.
348).

Hallam and Rachman (1972) stated that the accuracy of treatment
outcome predictions based on a cognitive dissonance theory of
aversion therapy depends on:

(1) The degree of volition of freedom that the S feels he has
in making counter-attitudinal statements and (2) the degree
of commitment to the counter-attitudinal statement or behaviour
(p. 348).

They added that the efficacy of treatment may be enhanced by
voluntary referral, belief in either the therapy or the therapist,
and "a high social cost of failing to benefit from treatment" (p.
348). This proposition was supported by Hallam et al.'s (1972)
finding that several alcoholic subjects in their nonaversion therapy group reported at follow-up that they were still abstaining
from drinking. Hence, cognitive dissonance and successful treatment outcome may have been due to their commitment to attend
psychotherapy sessions and receive in-patient hospital care.

INCUBATION OF FEAR AND COGNITIVE REHEARSAL

Two specific hypotheses have been advanced to explain the
generalization of therapeutic effects — Eysenck's (1968) "incubation of fear" hypothesis and Bandura's (1969) "cognitive rehearsal" hypothesis. The traditional consolidation-reminiscence theory
of incubation proposes that during the interval between CS-UCS
pairings, increased responsivity to the CS occurs because of consolidation of the memory trace. The conditioned response should
be maintained during extinction because of the increased responsivity, but as Eysenck (1968) stated, "consolidation is not expected to work over periods in excess of a few hours" (p. 311). Eysenck proposed an incubation theory that accounted for the long-
term resistance to extinction of conditioned responses. Eysenck
did not ignore the observation that extinction occurs when a CS
is presented in the absence of the UCS (designated as $\overline{CS}$ by Eysenck). He did, however, argue that presenting $\overline{CS}$ may also
lead to an increment in CR strength, so that:

The observed CR is the resultant of two opposing tendencies;
extinction will be observed if the decrementing tendencies are
greater than the incrementing ones, while *incubation* will be
observed if the incrementing tendencies are greater than the
decrementing ones (p. 312).

In developing his argument for incubation, Eysenck (1968) employed a concept that he called a nocive response (NR). Eysenck
explained this term:

A CS is followed by a UCS, say shock, which produces a
great variety of UCRs . . . . After a single pairing, or after
repeated pairings of CS and UCS, C̄S̄ produces some, or at
least segments of some, of the responses originally produced
by the UCS . . . . CS and C̄S̄ acquire the function of signal-
ling danger and coming pain, discomfort, fear and annoyance;
let us denote these nocive consequences as NRs (nocive responses) (p. 312).

In elaborating on this concept, Eysenck (1968) illustrated how incubation develops:

Shock is followed by pain, C̄S̄ is followed by fear. Shock +
CS is followed by fear + pain; this combined NR is more potent
(more disagreeable, more nocive, more aversive) than either
alone, and hence has greater reinforcing properties. C̄S̄ is
followed by fear as the CR, which is less reinforcing than
pain + fear, but may be sufficiently reinforcing to more than
counteract the decremental effects of extinction. When this
occurs, incubation takes place. When shock is experienced
a number of times, habituation/adaptation occurs. When shock
is accompanied by CS, the addition of fear to pain may delay
habituation/adaptation, or even become stronger in the balance and lead to the occurrence of NRs which are stronger
than the original UCR (p. 314).

Eysenck's theory, therefore, stresses the importance of the
strength of the UCR and CR rather than the strength of the UCS.
Strong UCRs are likely to produce incubation whereas weak UCRs
readily extinguish. Eysenck further argued that a strong UCS
does not necessarily produce a strong UCR and, conversely, that
a weak UCS may not result in a weak UCR. This implies that UCR
strength is not determined solely by UCS intensity. The following statement by Eysenck (1968) is based on this argument:

The UCS and UCR will of course usually be correlated, but
this correlation is far from perfect. Identical electric shocks
of medium intensity will have different effects on two people
of whom one is already terrified of electricity, while the other
is well accustomed to dealing with it; identical UCSs will lead
to quite different UCRs (p. 318).

In a more recent article, Eysenck (1979) again emphasized the role
of the UCR and CR:

The differentiation between UCS and UCR is in any case some-
what artificial from the point of view of the organism that is

being conditioned. Consider aversive conditioning, using shock. The shock is the UCS, and pain + fear the UCR; this makes sense from the point of view of the experimenter, who administers the UCS, while the S experiences the pain. However, the S does not feel shock (UCS) which produces pain (UCR); he experiences a painful shock, that is UCS and UCR are experienced simultaneously, and not as separate, consecutive entities. It is this Gestalt-like NR that is being linked with the CS through contiguity, and to which the CR eventually adds another increment of pain/fear which is introspectively very difficult or even impossible to differentiate from the original NR (p. 160).

Eysenck (1976, 1979) considered the strength of the UCS to be an important factor, however, in mediating incubation. He explained that incubation would not occur unless the UCS was initially strong enough to enable $\overline{CS}$ to overcome extinction. With regard to $\overline{CS}$ duration, Eysenck (1979) argued that "duration is important because the strength of the CR declines over time; the longer the exposure to $\overline{CS}$, the weaker will be the CR" (p. 162). The variable of $\overline{CS}$ duration, therefore, largely determines whether the net effect of $\overline{CS}$ will be incubation or extinction. To explain this, Eysenck has postulated the notion of a critical point of CR strength. If, at the time of $\overline{CS}$ termination, CR strength is above this critical point, enhancement of the CR (incubation) will occur. If CR strength is below the critical point at the time of $\overline{CS}$ termination, extinction will occur.

One writer (Bersh, 1980) has discussed Eysenck's theory in considerable detail. He noted that the amount of incubation or extinction increases as the difference between $\overline{CS}$ duration and the critical $\overline{CS}$ duration increases. As Bersh (personal communication) illustrated, "if the critical duration were 10 seconds, a 2-sec $\overline{CS}$ would increase the strength of the CR to a much greater extent than a 9-sec $\overline{CS}$, while a 20-sec $\overline{CS}$ would decrease CR strength to a much greater extent than an 11-sec $\overline{CS}$." Bersh added that the critical point theory provides no basis for "the *a priori* specification" of the critical point of CR strength. This point must be empirically determined for each subject. Once a particular $\overline{CS}$ duration has been shown empirically to increase CR strength, however, "further $\overline{CS}$ presentations with a duration no greater than this will produce additional increases in CR strength . . . . Similarly a $\overline{CS}$ duration shown to weaken the CR will continue to weaken it ever more rapidly" (Bersh, personal communication).

Bersh (1980) proposed that while the incubation theory provides a reasonable basis for enhancement of CR strength as a result of $\overline{CS}$, it has two major weaknesses:

1. Certain features of Eysenck's theory are contraindicated by data. These include the assumptions that the UCS in Pavlovian 'B' conditioning must elicit the *complete* UCR and that the CR must act as a drive. Fortunately, neither of these assumptions is actually important to the theory. The most fundamental requirement is that $\overline{CS}$ must elicit CR's (with accompanying stimuli) which remain sufficiently aversive at $\overline{CS}$ termination to reinforce the CS despite the intrinsic weakening effect of withholding the UCS.

2. A more serious defect of the theory involves its assumptions concerning CR strength as a function of UCS intensity and $\overline{CS}$ duration in relation to a critical level of strength . . . . Such functions determine the net reinforcement or extinction effect of $\overline{CS}$. These assumptions lead to the invalid deductions that extinction curves are *positively* decelerated and incubation curves *positively* accelerated. Most problematic for the theory is its lack of predictive power at its present stage of development. Since the outcome of $\overline{CS}$ is determined by antagonistic reinforcement and extinction processes, and since the theory does not permit a determination in advance of their relative strength, *any* laboratory or clinical result can be interpreted *post-facto*, but under the shadow of circularity (p. 16).

The significance of the "critical point" notion — based on the duration of $\overline{CS}$ exposure — is cogently illustrated in Eysenck's (1979) discussion of desensitization and flooding procedures. According to Eysenck (1979):

In . . . desensitization, the patient is protected against any strong anxiety arising during therapy by a procedure in which he is kept in a relaxed state, and is presented $\overline{CS}$, whether *in vivo* or in imagination, only at points on the hierarchy that will arouse him relatively little (i.e., points well below the critical point). If this point is ever exceeded, the $\overline{CS}$ is immediately withdrawn; it has often been demonstrated that when the critical point is reached or exceeded in desensitization, the success of treatment is imperilled, and the patient is actually made worse . . . . In flooding, on the other hand, the patient is immediately confronted with the most threatening $\overline{CS}$, that is one at the top of the hierarchy; this procedure, which includes explicitly an element of response prevention, is continued for periods of an hour or more. Both desensiti[z]ation and flooding are successful in practice . . . although they appear to proceed in contradictory directions . . . . The answer lies in the short duration of the exposure to high-anxiety $\overline{CS}$ which occurs in desensitization when the therapist makes an error; the critical point is exceeded, and consequently enhancement takes place, rather than extinction, which only occurs at levels of anxiety below the critical point. In flooding, exposure to the $\overline{CS}$ is continued long enough to get well below the critical point; hence extinction takes place, and no enhancement (p. 162).

On the basis of his theory, Eysenck (1979) predicted that a patient's problem would be exacerbated by flooding procedures that employed brief $\overline{CS}$ exposure time. Following this rationale, Eysenck suggested that if, in desensitization procedures, an exceptionally strong $\overline{CS}$ is inadvertently presented, the therapist should not withdraw the $\overline{CS}$ but should immediately employ a flooding procedure.

Quattlebaum has proposed an alternative explanation for an increment in CR strength during conditioning. His account was based primarily on the operant conditioning paradigm — that responses may be resistant to extinction because $\overline{CS}$ may provide negative reinforcement of an autonomic CR. In other words, on $\overline{CS}$ trials, the CR is not followed by (subject avoids) the aversive UCS. Quattlebaum (1970) illustrated this process:

On the first trial, the UCS is paired with the CS, eliciting the response, increase in blood pressure (BPR). Thus the sequence of events was clearly classical conditioning:

CS ------ UCS ------ UCR (BPR)

Note that there was no response following the CS. On the second trial the sequence of events was thus:

CS ------ CR (BPR)

Note that no event follows the response. It is possible that this trial contains elements of both operant and classical conditioning. The occurrence of the response was due to classical conditioning. The response was classically elicited, but the absence of the aversive stimulus (noncontingent though it may be) may be viewed as an operant avoidance paradigm. In other words, the organism failed to respond to the neutral stimulus (CS) on the first trial and was shocked; on the second trial, the organism responded and received no shock. Thus the previously neutral stimulus (CS) began to take on characteristics of a discriminative stimulus S^D in the presence of which BPR was followed by (noncontingent) absence of shock; in other words, noncontingent operant avoidance conditioning. This explanation would account for the extreme resistance to extinction, common to operant avoidance paradigms (p. 749).

The cognitive rehearsal hypothesis proposes that conditioned responses are maintained after therapy because:

A symbolic association between the deviant stimulus and the aversive UCS is strengthened every time thoughts about the treatment are triggered off by external stimuli (e.g., smell of alcohol) or when the patient voluntarily recalls treatment in order to control any remnants of his attraction to deviant objects (Hallam and Rachman, 1972, p. 349).

The incubation and rehearsal hypotheses differ, yet they similarly propose that "reexperiencing of the CS in real-life or the CS-UCS sequence in imagination is said to strengthen the association between the CS and the aversive response" (Hallam and Rachman, 1972, p. 349). Support for the cognitive rehearsal notion has been found by clinical workers (e.g., Laverty, 1966). Some clients in Laverty's study reported that whenever faced with a temptation to drink, they would recall the experiences they had during therapy. For example, one client reported that:

Whenever faced with a situation as to whether he should have a drink or not (which used to provide a degree of conflict in which alcohol was nearly always the winner) he gives as a way of getting out of the situation a graphic and detailed account of what he went through when he was treated with Scoline (Laverty, 1966, p. 655).

The results obtained in the Barlow, Leitenberg, and Agras (1969) research appear to weaken the cognitive rehearsal notion. These researchers found that sexually deviant subjects actually thought less about their habit after aversion therapy. In Laverty's (1966) study, support was found for the incubation of fear notion. Clients sometimes reported that their thoughts about treatment occurred spontaneously or that they had a "vivid re-experience of the actual traumatic episode, either in a dream or in a waking or semiwaking state. In these descriptions, the most common feature emphasized was a feeling described as fear" (Laverty, 1966, p.

654). Because there is evidence in favor of both the incubation and rehearsal hypotheses, it is difficult to determine which contributes more to the generalization of therapeutic effects.

STATE THEORY

Hallam and Rachman (1972) proposed a smale-scale state theory of aversion therapy which was also later discussed in their 1976 article "Current Status of Aversion Therapy." The schema of their theory, which remained essentially unchanged from 1972, is as follows:

1. During periods of altered responsiveness or sensitization, (to date, altered cardiac responsiveness) the target behavior is suppressed.
2. Sensitization can be induced by electrical aversion therapy, other behavioral means, or by a range of nonspecific clinical or nonclinical events (e.g., discovery, arrest, drugs, family pressure, psychiatric influences, etc.).
3. The effects of sensitization (e.g., cardiac responsivity) will diminish in time.
3a. A rapid decline is associated with therapeutic failure.
3b. A slow decline is associated with therapeutic success.
4. Although response-contingent punishment training schedules are not an essential prerequisite, their use will facilitate the suppression of the deviant behavior.
5. If during the period of sensitization the behavior is adequately suppressed, then two factors will help maintain the change: the development of alternative, reinforcing behavior and/or the reinforcement derived from the success in suppressing the target behavior itself (Hallam and Rachman, 1976, p. 217).

Although Hallam and Rachman's state theory is empirically testable, they asserted that:

The main problems of the schema are its lack of specificity (e.g., which measures indicate sensitization) and the certainty of finding complicated exceptions (Hallam and Rachman, 1976, p. 218).

TWO-FACTOR THEORY

Two-factor theory is perhaps the most popular explanation of aversive control. As stated by Seligman and Johnston (1973), two-factor theory's account of punishment and avoidance learning is embodied in two tenets:

1. By classical conditioning, when a CS is paired with an aversive UCS (such as shock), the CS comes to elicit the conditioned response of fear.
2. Fear motivates the avoidance response. When the response is made, the CS terminates, fear is reduced, and the avoidance response is reinforced by this fear reduction (p. 70).

The first factor in avoidance learning is the acquisition of the fear response by Pavlovian conditioning and the second factor is the instrumental learning of an avoidance response via fear reduction.

In his chapter on "Punishment and Fear," Adams (1976) enumerated six assumptions of two-factor theory:

1. Pain is an innate response of the autonomic nervous system.
2. Pain can be conditioned to any stimulus. The aspect of the pain response that is conditioned to a stimulus is called fear (sometimes it is called anxiety). The learning of fear is by classical conditioning.
3. Fear is motivating.
4. Fear has cue (stimulus) properties which are called response-produced stimuli.
5. Response-produced stimuli can become the cue for any response through learning.
6. The reduction of the fear motivation is a basis for instrumental learning (pp. 124-125).

Mowrer (1947) regarded negative emotional conditioning as the problem-making aspect of avoidance learning and the instrumental process as the problem-solving aspect. Figure 28 illustrates Mowrer's two-factor theory. Conceptually, instrumental avoidance learning is similar to escape learning. This assumption can be made on the basis of two types of behavior exhibited during training; that is, (a) escape from the UCS early in training and (b) escape from the CS later in training. Wahlsten and Cole (1972) regarded CS-escape as being "reinforcement of avoidance by response-termination of a fear-eliciting CS" (p. 381). Another writer (Schwartz, 1978) has also explained the acquisition of the

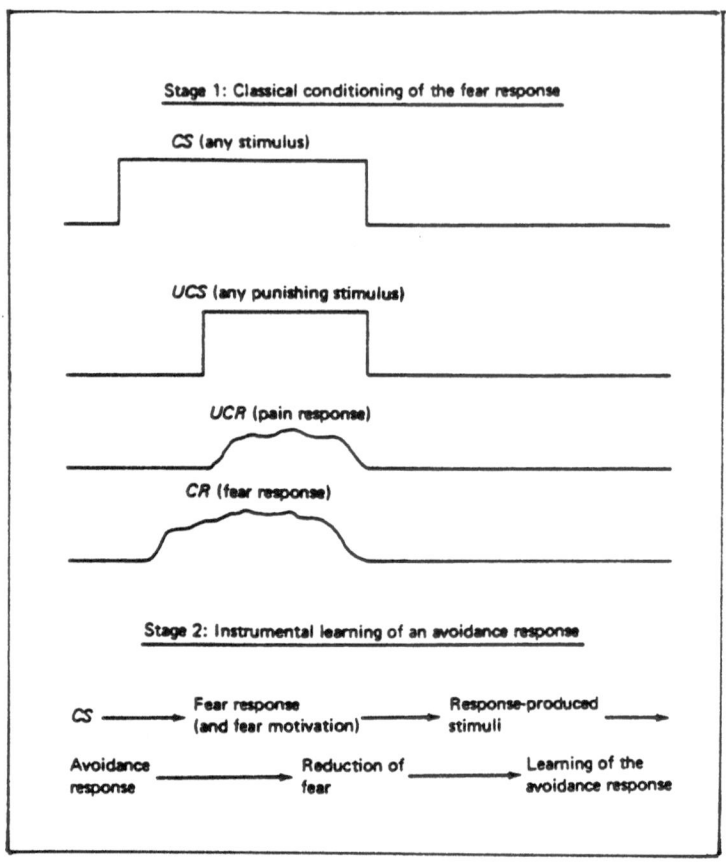

Figure 28. The stages of Mowrer's two-factor theory. Fear is learned in Stage 1 by classical conditioning, and avoidance behavior is instrumentally learned in Stage 2 when it produces fear reduction. From *Learning and memory: An introduction*, by J. A. Adams. Homewood, Il.: Dorsey Press, 1976, p. 125.

avoidance response in terms of instrumental escape learning:

> First, the animal learns to escape the shock. While escape is occurring, however, Pavlovian conditioning is also occurring; on each trial, tone (CS) is paired with shock (US). After a number of trials, the tone should elicit fear just as the shock does. The animal may now make the escape response to escape from the fearful CS. But escape from the CS is avoid-

ance of the US. Thus the two-factor theory of avoidance suggests that avoidance is not really avoidance at all. It is escape from a stimulus which, through pairing with shock, has
become fear-provoking. Notice how elegantly two-factor
theory solves the problem mentioned earlier of having a non-
event (the absence of shock) maintain avoidance; it is not the
absence of shock at all, but the elimination of the CS, which
maintains avoidance. Similarly, since escape is crucial to
successful avoidance behavior, the theory maintains that both
Pavlovian and operant factors influence and maintain avoidance (p. 251).

Similarly, Seligman and Johnston (1973) have noted that two-factor theory dismisses the anticipatory aspect of avoidance learning:

Rather than responding to ward off a shock in the future, an
"avoider" is actually escaping from fear-evoking stimuli in the
present [CS] (p. 70).

The Pavlovian and instrumental components of the two-factor
theory of avoidance learning were separately illustrated in a classic study by Brown and Jacobs. Two groups of rats were used –
a fear group and a control group. During training, rats in the
fear group were given 10 inescapable buzzer-shock presentations
in an enclosed box on each of 4 consecutive days. The control
group was trained in basically the same way, except that "no
shocks were given the controls at any time" (Brown and Jacobs,
1949, p. 749). In the second phase of the experiment, a barrier
was introduced to the box and the rats were permitted to escape
the CS by jumping over the barrier into a second compartment.
Only the buzzer CS was presented on these trials. Brown and
Jacobs (1949) observed that "experimental animals [fear group]
exhibited a progressive decrease in the latency of the barrier-
crossing response with successive non-shock trials" (p. 750).
Controls did not learn the jumping response. Brown and Jacobs
(1949) concluded that reduction of the classically conditioned fear
to the buzzer CS functioned to reinforce the learning of the instrumental barrier-jumping response.

According to two-factor theory, the number of CS-UCS pairings influences the amount of fear that is learned. To demonstrate this relationship, Kalish (1954) presented either 1, 3, 9, or
27 CS-UCS pairings to different groups of rats. After receiving
the stipulated number of pairings of the compound light-buzzer
CS and inescapable shock in an enclosed box, the animals were

placed in a two-compartment box in which they were presented
with CS-only trials. They could terminate the fear-arousing CS
by jumping over a barrier into a second compartment. Kalish
(1954) found that the greater the number of CS-UCS pairings,
the more quickly the avoidance response was learned on nonshock
trials.

Critique of Two-Factor Theory

Seligman and Johnston (1973) have reviewed several criticisms of the two-factor theory of avoidance learning. Two of these
pertained to (a) problems in accounting for resistance to extinction and (b) problems in specifying CSs.

Problems in Accounting for Resistance to Extinction

According to two-factor theory, an avoidance response should
readily extinguish during standard extinction procedures. Seligman and Johnston (1973) have outlined the predicted sequence of
events:

> On those trials in which a response occurs in the presence of
> the CS, no shock occurs. So, we have a Pavlovian extinction
> trial: the fear-evoking CS complex is paired with no shock.
> Fear to the CS should decrease monotonically, and extinction
> of the response in the presence of the CS should take place
> at about the rate of the Pavlovian fear extinction. After sev-
> eral dozen occurrences of the CS without the US, fear should
> be reduced to near zero. If the central state motivating the
> response were Pavlovian . . . avoidance would extinguish
> rapidly (pp. 80-81).

Avoidance responding, however, is highly resistant to standard
extinction procedures, an observation which poses a problem for
two-factor theory. Seligman and Johnston (1973) have proposed
that the concepts of safety signal reinforcement and automatization
may assist two-factor theory in circumventing this problem. The
safety signal reinforcement hypothesis claims that during acquisition, external CS termination and the internal feedback from performing the avoidance response become safety signals because they
have been paired with no shock. These safety signals function
to reinforce avoidance responding. Seligman and Johnston argued
that during extinction, safety signals continue to reinforce the
avoidance response. They noted one problem, however, that accompanies the safety signal reinforcement hypothesis when it is

applied to two-factor theory's account of avoidance learning. Because this hypothesis proposes that avoidance responding is not
maintained by fear, it cannot adequately explain extinction by response blocking procedures. In fact, it directly contradicts the
classical conditioning component of two-factor theory which proposes that during response blocking procedures, the avoidance
response is extinguished because fear to the CS is extinguished.
This conflict between the safety signal hypothesis and two-factor
theory in accounting for extinction by response blocking has been
cogently stated by Seligman and Johnston (1973):

> If it is only the positive reinforcement of the response pro-
> vided by a safety signal which maintains avoidance, and fear
> has dropped out, there is no fear CR to be extinguished (p.
> 85).

In summary, it appears that the safety signal hypothesis can assist two-factor theory in explaining the resistance of avoidance
responding to standard extinction procedures but it does not contribute to an explanation of extinction by response blocking.

According to the principle of automatization, well learned responses come to be initiated without motivational antecedents (Kimble and Perlmuter, in Seligman and Johnston, 1973, p. 85). Like
the safety signal reinforcement hypothesis, automatization allows
two-factor theory to adequately account for resistance to extinction but it is weak in explaining extinction by response blocking.
This point was illustrated in a study conducted nearly 3 decades
ago (Miller, 1951). In Phase 1 of Miller's experiment, rats learned
to escape shock by running from one compartment to another in
a two-compartment box. In Phase 2, they were returned to the
first compartment on each trial but were not shocked. The door
between the two compartments was closed and could only be opened by a wheel-turning response. After exhibiting a number of
symptoms of fear such as urination and defecation and performing
a variety of goal-directed responses, the rats eventually learned
the wheel-turning response. The speed of operating the wheel
increased on subsequent trials despite the absence of shock. Phase
3 of the experiment was designed so that a bar-press response
opened the door. Miller (1951) observed that the subjects abandoned the wheel-turning response and learned to open the door
by pressing the bar. Hence, the emitting of a particular avoidance response such as wheel-turning cannot be regarded as an
automated sequence of actions with no motivational antecedents.
The rats had learned to fear the first compartment which in turn
motivated the learning of the avoidance responses of wheel-turning

and bar-pressing. It seems, therefore, that the principle of automatization offers only minimal support for a two-factor theory account of extinction by response blocking.

Problems in Specifying CSs

Another weakness of two-factor theory is in identifying the
fear-eliciting CS in certain types of conditioning paradigms (Seligman and Johnston, 1973). In trace conditioning, for example, it
is unlikely that the external CS itself elicits the instrumental
avoidance response because the CS may be terminated *before* the
response is emitted (see Figure 29). This being the case, it follows that external CS termination cannot function to reinforce
avoidance responding through fear reduction.

Seligman and Johnston (1973) suggested that this proposed
theoretical weakness of two-factor theory may be partially overcome by considering the plausibility of internal rather than external CSs. They posited that in trace conditioning, two types
of internal CSs may be functionally equivalent to an external CS.
The first is the memory trace of the external CS and the second
is the proprioceptive and kinesthetic feedback from not having
performed the appropriate avoidance response. The feedback
from *inappropriate* responding would be associated with the UCS
and would therefore acquire the fear-arousing attributes of an external CS. On the other hand, the internal feedback from performing the *appropriate* avoidance response would be associated

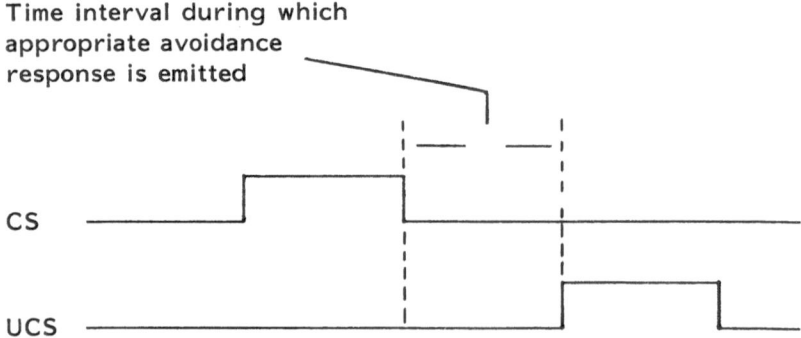

Figure 29. Temporal relation of avoidance response to external CS
in trace conditioning. In this illustration, the CS is terminated before the avoidance response is emitted.

with the absence of the UCS and should result in fear reduction. In turn, fear reduction should reinforce avoidance responding. Other researchers (for instance, Rescorla and Solomon, 1967) have also suggested that internal CSs function to motivate and re- inforce avoidance responding. In relating this point to two-factor theory's account of avoidance learning, Rescorla and Solomon (1967) stated:

> The pairing of a CS with electric shock leads to the develop- ment of a conditioned "fear" reaction. Increase in sensory feedback from that "fear" reaction is postulated to instigate the instrumental avoidance response while reduction in the feedback rewards it (p. 166).

It has been argued and shown by several investigators (e.g., Kamin, 1956) that CS termination is not a necessary condition for establishing avoidance behavior. A review of some of the salient features of Kamin's research is in order. He summarized, as fol- lows, the four conditions in his study:

> The groups were: the "Normal" Ss, which by responding could both terminate the CS and avoid the US; the "Termi- nate-CS" Ss, which could *only* terminate the CS; the "Avoid- US" Ss, which could *only* avoid the US; and the "Classical" Ss, which could neither terminate the CS nor avoid the US (Kamin, 1956, p. 420).

The procedure involved presenting a buzzer CS followed 5 seconds after its onset by a shock UCS. If the rat did not run from the shocked compartment of the experimental box during the 5 sec- onds, the UCS was presented and both the CS and UCS continued until the animal ran from the box. These trials were termed "es- cape" trials. If, however, the animal ran from the first compart- ment after CS onset but before the onset of the shock, the trial was termed a "CR" trial. For CR trials, the consequence of the running response differed for each group. For the Normal group, the CS was terminated and the UCS avoided; for the Terminate- CS group, the CS was terminated but the UCS was presented ac- cording to schedule; for the Avoid-UCS group, the CS continued for 5 seconds but the UCS was not presented; for the Classical group, the response had no effect on either the CS or the UCS.

The subjects in the Normal group emitted CRs more frequent- ly and with shorter latencies than the subjects in the other three groups. Statistical analysis revealed the difference in fre- quency to be statistically significant. There were no significant differences among the other groups. The number of "CRs" emitted by the Avoid-UCS subjects, however, was greater than for either the Classical or Terminate-CS groups. This may have been due to the similarity between the procedures for the Normal and Avoid-UCS groups. Like the Normal subjects, the Avoid-UCS subjects could avoid the aversive stimulus by emitting the appropriate response. Although they could not terminate the CS, Kamin (1956) has explained how CS offset may have reinforced avoidance responding for the subjects in the Avoid-UCS condition:

> The Avoid-US rats *do*, in effect, terminate the CS — though termination of the CS is delayed for a few seconds. Thus, if a rat in this group responded to the CS with a latency of, e.g., 3 sec, its CR was followed by termination of the CS in only 2 sec. This slightly delayed reward ought to reinforce responding (p. 423).

Because both groups that could avoid the UCS (Normal and Avoid-UCS) responded with more CRs than the two groups that could not avoid the UCS (Terminate-CS and Classical), it appears that the salient factor in avoidance learning was UCS avoidance and not CS termination. The finding that the Avoid-UCS subjects (who could not terminate the CS) ranked second in percent of "CRs" emitted weakens two-factor theory's claim that CS termination is necessary for avoidance learning. Seligman and Johnston (1973) have argued, however, that Kamin's study did not meet the fear reduction requirements of two-factor theory. Concerning the Classical group and the Terminate-CS group, Seligman and Johnston stated:

> The paradigm of CS-escape with noncontingent delivery of USs cannot meet the reinforcement requirements of fear theory. By definition, if US presentation is noncontingent, the stimuli facing an animal after r [responding] and r̄ [not responding] will lead to shock with equal probabilities and will be equally fear provoking. So fear reduction contingent on r will not occur (p. 74).

In Sidman (free operant) avoidance learning, performing the appropriate response postpones the onset of the UCS. The presentation of the UCS can therefore be indefinitely postponed if the subject's response is the appropriate one and if interresponse times are consistently shorter than the response-UCS interval. If the appropriate response is not emitted, the UCS is presented at fixed time intervals. Because no external CS is presented in Sidman avoidance, Seligman and Johnston (1973) proposed that fear is elicited by an internal compound CS which consists of:

Feedback from not having made the response . . . together
with the length of time since the preceding response (Seligman and Johnston, 1973, p. 71).

Another writer (Schwartz, 1978) has similarly elaborated on the
fear-eliciting CS in Sidman avoidance:

If the US occurs at regular intervals, then the passage of a
certain amount of time can become a CS and elicit responses.
This temporal conditioning may well be occurring in free-
operant avoidance procedures. Time between a response
and shock is constant, and one could easily imagine that fear
could be conditioned to a period of time after the last response. When the organism made a response, fear would be
low or nonexistent. As time passed without a response, fear
would grow. When it became sufficiently intense, the response would occur, escaping the fear and as a by-product
avoiding the shock. There is ample evidence that animals
that learn to avoid shocks on shock-postponement procedures
do not distribute their res[p]onses randomly in time; rather,
the likelihood of a response increases as the time since the
last response increases (p. 251).

BIOLOGICAL THEORY

Theories of avoidance learning have tended to favor the proposition that an animal initially escapes from an aversive UCS and,
because of classically conditioned fear to the CS, eventually learns
to emit the appropriate instrumental avoidance response. Because
animals *rapidly* learn to avoid danger in the natural environment,
biological theorists claim that this formulation is not adequate.
Bolles (1970) contended that in the face of danger, an animal will
respond with species-specific defense reactions (SSDRs). Freezing, attacking, and fleeing are three common SSDRs. These responses are selected by the animal according to some innate hier-
archical scale until one of them enables the danger to be avoided.
In the laboratory setting, Bolles (1970) proposed that an animal
will quickly learn to avoid a noxious stimulus if the required response is similar to an SSDR. For example, if jumping out of a
box is the required response for a rat, it may quickly learn to
avoid the UCS. Conversely, an animal will learn slowly or not at
all if the required avoidance response does not resemble an SSDR.
If the response is a lever-press, for example, a rat may never
learn to avoid the UCS unless he accidentally freezes on the lever.

Schwartz (1978) explained that "only when all of the animal's de-
fensive repertoire has been sampled and proven ineffective will
non-SSDRs occur" (p. 262). According to biological theory,
therefore, the topography of the required avoidance response determines the rate of avoidance learning.

COGNITIVE THEORY

Seligman and Johnston (1973) have proposed a cognitive
theory of avoidance learning that was conceptualized within the
framework of F. W. Irwin's cognitive theory of behavior. Emotional and cognitive aspects of avoidance learning were included
in Seligman and Johnston's theory. The cognitive component of
the theory proposed that outcome preference and the learning of
response-outcome expectancies were crucial to avoidance learning.
For a procedure employing a faradic stimulus, the assumed preference and outcome expectancies are outlined in the following five-
point summary:

1. A subject prefers no shock to shock.
2. A subject learns two expectancies during avoidance conditioning. One of these is that shock will not be presented if the appropriate response is emitted within a given
   period of time. This time interval is specified by the CS-
   UCS interval in signalled shock and by the R-S interval
   in unsignalled shock.
3. The second learned expectancy is that shock will occur
   if the appropriate response is not made within a stipulated
   time interval.
4. These two expectancies are strengthened when they are
   confirmed and weakened when disconfirmed. For instance,
   the expectancy that a particular response will not be followed by shock is confirmed when shock does not follow
   the emitted response. This expectancy is weakened if the
   selected response is made but is followed by shock (see
   Table 1).

Similarly, the expectancy that responding inappropriately during the CS-UCS interval will be followed by shock is confirmed if
the subject does not respond appropriately and is shocked. This
expectancy is weakened if the animal is not shocked for responding
inappropriately during the CS-UCS interval, as schematized in
Table 2.

TABLE 1. Effect of Response Outcome on Subject's Learned Expectation Related to Emitting an Appropriate Avoidance Response

Expectation	Behavior	Observed outcome	Expectation confirmed / disconfirmed
No shock if AR emitted during CS-UCS interval	AR emitted during CS-UCS interval	No shock	Confirmed
		Shock	Disconfirmed

Note: AR = avoidance response.

  5. The probability that the avoidance response will be emitted increases monotonically as the two expectancies are repeatedly confirmed.

The emotional component of Seligman and Johnston's (1973) theory is based on the notion that responses are elicited by classically conditioned fear. Fear reduction, however, plays no role in the theory's explanation of avoidance learning. The postulates of the emotional component of Seligman and Johnston's theory are:

  1. Fear is classically conditioned to a CS paired with shock.
  2. Fear is classically extinguished to the CS when the CS is not followed by shock.

TABLE 2. Effect of Response Outcome on Subject's Learned Expectation Related to Emitting an Inappropriate Avoidance Response

Expectation	Behavior	Observed outcome	Expectation confirmed / disconfirmed
Shock if AR not emitted during CS-UCS interval	AR not emitted during CS-UCS interval	Shock	Confirmed
		No shock	Disconfirmed

Note: AR = avoidance response.

3. Fear can be indexed by autonomic responses and skeletal responses elicited by the CS. These skeletal responses may, with some probability, include the specified avoidance response or similar responses (p. 94).

Seligman and Johnston asserted that the emotional component of their theory explains the acquisition of an avoidance response and that the cognitive component accounts for response maintenance. They have used elements of biological theory to account for the learning of an avoidance response. Not only does a fear-evoking CS facilitate avoidance learning, but the avoidance response is more readily learned if it resembles one of the animal's SSDRs, that is, if it is already in the animal's natural escape response repertoire. In relating this point to cognitive theory, Seligman and Johnston added that learning is facilitated when the topographies of the SSDR and the required avoidance response are similar because the "avoidance response emitted-no aversive stimulus" expectancy is confirmed early in training. Once avoidance responses begin to occur and expectancies begin to be confirmed, the cognitive aspect of the theory takes over.

Cognitive theory adequately explains the resistance of avoidance responding to extinction by standard procedures. Since the animal has learned during training that emitting the appropriate avoidance response to the CS will be followed by "no shock," it is reasonable that the subject will continue to emit the same response when the CS is presented during Pavlovian extinction trials. Cognitive theory does not encounter problems in explaining the effectiveness of response blocking techniques in eliminating avoidance behavior. When the animal is prevented from responding during CS-no shock trials, it learns to associate not responding with the absence of shock. This in turn disconfirms and weakens the "no response-shock" expectation that was learned during avoidance training.

Seligman and Johnston (1973) have asserted that, unlike two-factor theory, their cognitive theory maintains that "*response extinction* occurs independently of Pavlovian *fear extinction*" (p. 93). They stated that in response blocking, it is possible that the CS still evokes fear in the animal despite the observation that the motoric avoidance response has extinguished.

5

Personality and Conditionability

PAVLOV'S THEORY

Pavlov (1927) proposed that when stimuli are detected by an organism's sensory receptors, the excitation is conveyed to the cortex where excitatory neurons are activated. An excitatory neural pattern is established when a stimulus is repeatedly presented to an organism. When two stimuli are repeatedly presented, the neural patterns enable the organism to predict the presentation of one stimulus from the occurrence of the other. This explanation seemed to satisfactorily account for the conditioning of a salivary response to a buzzer by dogs in Pavlov's experiments. Inhibitory neurons in the cortex act to depress the excitatory cells and, therefore, interfere with establishing and maintaining positively conditioned reflexes.

During his investigations, Pavlov found conditionability and temperament to be highly correlated. He specifically observed that normally active, friendly dogs did not readily form conditioned reflexes. Paradoxically, they became drowsy and fell asleep during training. Pavlov (1927) postulated that this type of dog's cortical processes were predominantly excitatory, thereby requiring novel and varied stimuli to maintain the arousal necessary for conditioning. The monotony of the conditioning procedure quickly exhausted the dog's excitatory cells and, therefore, interfered with conditioning. Dogs of this "extreme excitatory" temperament were found to be readily conditioned when a constant succession of novel stimuli was available during the conditioning procedure (Pavlov, 1927, p. 287). On the other hand, dogs that appeared afraid and inhibited in their natural environment conditioned well, once familiar with the apparatus and the investigator. Inhibitory cortical processes predominate in this type of dog. Pavlov re-

107

ported, however, that only conditioned inhibitory reflexes were stable and strongly established in this "extreme inhibitory" type of dog. By inhibitory reflex, Pavlov meant learning *not* to respond to the unreinforced stimulus in a compound CS.

Between these two extreme excitatory and inhibitory temperaments, Pavlov (1928) postulated two balanced types. The first type possessed a well established balance between excitation and inhibition. According to Pavlov, this type of dog resembled the extreme excitatory dog in behavioral characteristics but not in conditionability. Both positive and inhibitory reflexes were readily formed. The second type represented a balance between excitatory and inhibitory processes that was not stable. Conditioned reflexes were easily established but not strongly maintained. Pavlov stated that the behavior but not the conditionability of this second balanced temperament type resembled that of the extreme inhibitory animal.

In addition to relating temperament to conditionability, Pavlov (1928) equated his four nervous system types to the four personality types identified by the classical temperament theory of Hippocrates and Galen. A recent writer (Monte, 1977, pp. 605-606) has summarized this relationship:

Extreme Excitatory Type: Choleric (Poor conditionability)

Extreme Inhibitory Type: Melancholic (Good inhibitory
                                  conditionability)

Balanced (Excitatory) Type: Sanguine (Good conditionability)

Balanced (Inhibitory) Type: Phlegmatic (Good [conditionabil-
                                  ity] but easily distracted)

EYSENCK'S PERSONALITY CLASSIFICATION

Eysenck (1957), like Pavlov, believed that the source of the observable differences in the four personality types was in the inhibitory and excitatory processes of the nervous system. Eysenck felt, however, that human behavior could be better described by adapting the four humoral types of classical temperament theory to a two-dimensional classification of personality. The two dimensions underlying Eysenck's description of personality were introversion/extraversion and stability/unstability. Eysenck's classification of personality is illustrated in Figure 30.

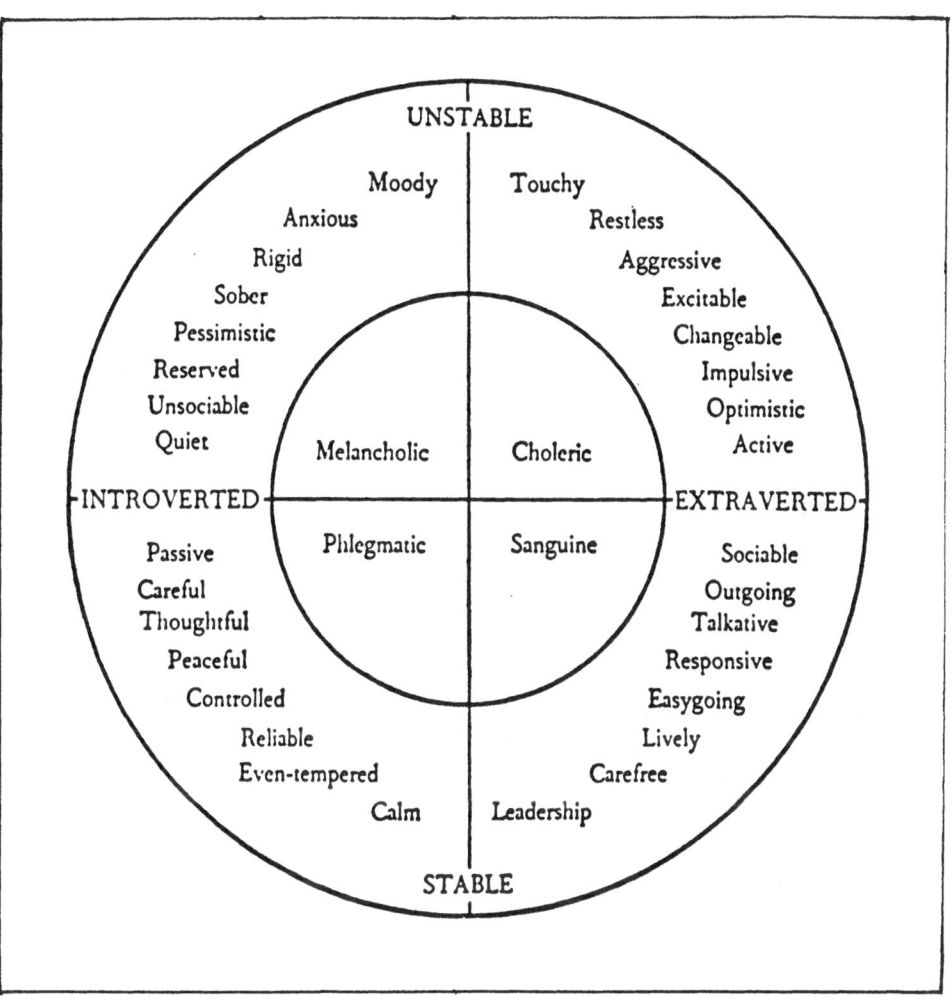

Figure 30. The diagram shows Galen's medieval personality theory of the four temperaments (inner circle) and the results of modern experimental and statistical studies of personality structure (outer circle). From *Crime and personality*, by H. J. Eysenck. London: Paladin, 1970, p. 51.

DIFFERENCES BETWEEN PAVLOV'S AND EYSENCK'S CLASSIFICATIONS

Monte (1977) has summarized the differences between Eysenck's and Pavlov's classifications of personality types as they relate to classical temperaments. This is depicted in Table 3. Although Eysenck's (1957) classification of personality differed from Pavlov's, the concepts of inhibition and excitation nonetheless figured prominently in his theory. Eysenck assumed that individuals with phlegmatic and melancholic temperaments possess extremely sensitive excitation processes which cause them to withdraw from environmental stimulation. It was on this basis that Eysenck classified melancholic and phlegmatic types as introverts. The distinctive feature of the sanguine and choleric personalities, according to Eysenck, is their responsiveness and attentiveness to their surroundings. He proposed, therefore, that these two personality types have highly inhibitory cortical processes and that they constantly seek environmental stimulation to overcome this cortical inertia. Eysenck (1957) classified the sanguine and choleric personalities as extroverts.

STRONG AND WEAK NERVOUS SYSTEMS

Gray (1967) has reviewed the research of Teplov who, like Eysenck, applied Pavlov's inhibition/excitation theory to man. Teplov's research focused primarily on excitation and specifically on the differences between strong and weak excitatory processes; that is, between strong and weak nervous systems. The following statement, made by Gray in an earlier publication (Gray, 1964), outlines the differences:

> The weak nervous system is more *sensitive* than the strong: it begins to respond at stimulus intensities which are ineffective for the strong nervous system; throughout the stimulus-intensity continuum its responses are closer to its maximum level of responding than the responses of the strong nervous system; and it displays its maximum response, or the response decrement which follows this maximum, at lower stimulus intensities than the strong nervous system.
> These same differences may be expressed by saying that the strong nervous system is more *stable* than the weak — it is better able to withstand extreme intensities of stimulation, better able to continue responding appropriately and without decrement at high stimulus intensities (p. 281).

TABLE 3. Pavlov's Types and Eysenck's Dimensions Contrasted

Classical temperaments	Pavlov's types	Behavioral traits (Pavlov)	Eysenck's dimensions	Classical temperaments
Choleric	Extreme excitatory	Outgoing, affable friendly at liberty, but becomes drowsy in monotony of experimental chamber. Conditions well only when stimuli are varied and novel. Neurosis caused by failure of inhibition and resembles human *psychasthenia*.	Extreme emotional introvert (neurotic)	Melancholic
Melancholic	Extreme inhibitory	Cowardly, cringing, nervous, this dog conditions well in the monotony of the experiment. But positive reflexes (e.g., salivation to reinforced stimulus) are poorer than negative conditioned reflexes (e.g., withholding response, or discrimination). Neurosis caused by failure of excitatory cells and resembles human *hysteria*.	Extreme emotional extrovert (neurotic)	Choleric
Sanguine	Balanced excitatory	Conditions well in both positive and negative responses. Outgoing, affable, like extreme excitatory type. Resists experimental neurosis.	Stable introvert	Phlegmatic
Phlegmatic	Balanced inhibitory	Conditions well, but positive responses disrupted easily. Quiet, stolid, and alert, like inhibitory animal when calm. Resists experimental neurosis.	Stable extrovert	Sanguine

Note reversal of classical temperaments between Eysenck's and Pavlov's schemes. Furthermore, the behavioral descriptions are Pavlov's, *not* Eysenck's, and in fact contradict Eysenck's trait descriptions of introverted and extroverted personalities. Based on Pavlov, 1928, p. 377; Pavlov, 1927, p. 286; Eysenck, 1957; Teplov, 1964, pp. 13, 18. From *Beneath the Mask: An Introduction to Theories of Personality*, by C. F. Monte. New York: Praeger, 1977, pp. 610-611.

Eysenck (1973a) has pointed out a parallel between the concepts of strong and weak nervous systems and the notions of introversion and extraversion. He postulated that the "'weak' personality type appears to resemble the introvert, the 'strong' personality type the extravert" (p. 156).

RELATION OF INTROVERSION-EXTROVERSION TO
SENSORY THRESHOLDS AND PAIN TOLERANCE

Eysenck (1967) asserted that introverts should demonstrate
lower sensory thresholds than extroverts because of the sensitiv-
ity of their weak nervous systems to stimulation. Haslam has reported significantly lower pain thresholds for introverts than for
extroverts and Smith found lower auditory thresholds among introverts (in Eysenck, 1967). In addition, Eysenck claimed that
pain tolerance should be negatively correlated with neuroticism-
introversion and positively related to extroversion (Lynn and Eysenck, 1961). This prediction was based on findings that extroverts develop inhibition more quickly and dissipate it more slowly
than introverts. It follows that pain sensations should be inhibited more quickly and strongly in extroverts. Another factor that
indicates greater pain tolerance for extroverts is their poorer conditionability. As Beecher (in Lynn and Eysenck, 1961) stated,
extroverts should not develop the conditioned fear response which
accompanies and summates with physiological pain to the same extent as introverts. Eysenck (in Lynn and Eysenck, 1961) subjected introverts and extroverts to heat-pain stimulation. They
were instructed to tolerate the pain for as long as possible, up to
a 20-second time limit. Pain tolerance ranged from 17.2 seconds
for highly extroverted subjects to 5.6 seconds for subjects low on
the extroversion scale. Eight of the highly extroverted subjects
reached the 20-second time limit while *none* of the most introverted
subjects did. Hall and Stride (in Lynn and Eysenck, 1961) also
found that among psychiatric patients, pain tolerance was lowest
for introverted neurotics. These findings supported Eysenck's
hypothesis concerning the relation of pain threshold and pain tolerance to the personality dimensions of introversion and extroversion.
    Weak and strong nervous systems both function with a protec-
tive threshold that Pavlov called the threshold of transmarginal
inhibition (Gray, 1964, pp. 161-162). A conditioned response increases in magnitude as stimulus intensity increases, but at the
point of transmarginal inhibition (TMI), the conditioned response

decreases in magnitude or ceases altogether. Although the weak
nervous system of the introvert is activated at lower levels of
stimulation than the strong nervous system of the extrovert, a
weak system also "shuts down" at lower levels of stimulation. As
Eysenck stated in his 1967 publication, "the weaker the nervous
system the earlier both thresholds [sensory and transmarginal in-
hibition] are reached" (p. 242). Figure 31 illustrates the different effects of stimulus intensity on the conditioned responses of
individuals with strong and weak nervous systems.

REACTIVE AND CONDITIONED INHIBITION

Conditioned responses are also affected by two types of inhibition, reactive and conditioned inhibition (Hull, in Eysenck, 1967,
1970). These variables affect an organism's drive level and previous habit strengths. A minor digression is required to outline

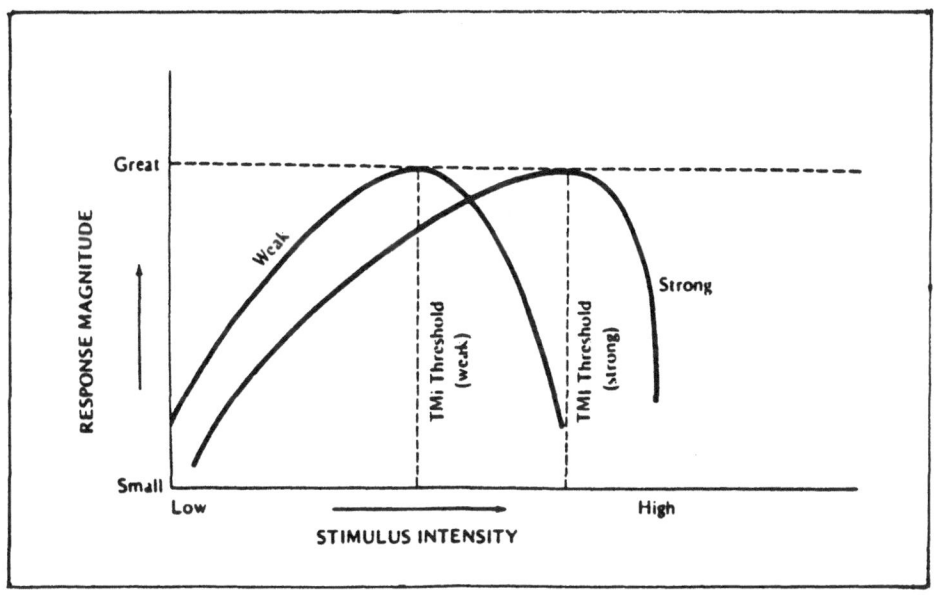

Figure 31. Transmarginal inhibition (TMI) thresholds for weak
and strong nervous systems. From *Beneath the mask: An introduction to theories of personality*, by C. F. Monte. New York:
Praeger, 1977, p. 613.

selected aspects of Hull's theory. Although Hull's formulation was developed to explain the processes involved in instrumental conditioning, the concepts of inhibition and excitation are central to the theory. Hull's basic premise was that learning will not occur unless a drive is present and unless that drive is reduced (Bugelski, 1971). If a stimulus is followed by a response which in turn is reinforced by drive reduction, the association between the stimulus and response is strengthened. The strength of the association between a stimulus and a response was termed *habit strength* by Hull. This term was denoted as $_SH_R$. The likelihood that a learned response will be made at any given moment was called reaction potential and was depicted as $_SE_R$. Reaction potential was considered to be a function of drive (D) and habit strength ($_SH_R$). D has to activate $_SH_R$ in order for the learned response to occur. Even if habit strength were high, the learned response would not be emitted without D (Hergenhahn, 1976). For example, if an animal has learned a lever-press response in order to obtain food, it would subsequently press the lever *only* when it was hungry. Observable performance, therefore, is a function of (a) how often the response was rewarded in a particular situation, and (b) the extent to which drive is present. This functional relationship was depicted mathematically by Hull as:

$$_SE_R = {}_SH_R \times D$$

Hull postulated that with repeated responding, fatigue, or reactive inhibition (I_R) builds up cumulatively until it is sufficiently strong to inhibit further action (Bugelski, 1971, p. 76). Subsequent cessation of responding leads to dissipation of the reactive inhibition and hence to a reduction of the negative drive of fatigue. This in turn produces conditioned inhibition, which is symbolized as $_SI_R$. That is, since not responding is rewarded by relief from fatigue, the organism develops a conditioned negative habit of not responding. Both types of inhibition "operate *against* the elicitation of a learned response and are therefore subtracted from reaction potential" (Hergenhahn, 1976, p. 135). Effective reaction potential ($_S\bar{E}_R$), therefore, is depicted by the following equation:

$$_S\bar{E}_R = (D \times {}_SH_R) - (I_R + {}_SI_R)$$

At the same time, however, they are functionally different. Reactive inhibition, an innate negative drive, predictably dissipates with time; conditioned inhibition, a learned negative habit, is relatively stable.

Eysenck (1970) applied the Hullian concepts of drive, inhibition, and habit strength to human performance:

The stronger the drive, and the more highly developed the
habits which are necessary for carrying out . . . a task, the
better . . . [the] performance will be. . . . . If a person is
carrying out a task, particularly under conditions of massed
practice, then inhibition will continue to accumulate. Being
a negative drive, it will subtract from the positive drive under which the organism is working. And, finally, when inhibition builds up to such an extent that it is equal to the
positive drive under which the person is working, he will
simply cease to work altogether, because now drive is equal
to inhibition, and drive minus inhibition equals zero (pp. 84-
85).

The cessation of activity may be only momentary but, nonetheless,
Eysenck (1970) predicted that it would occur. Eysenck called
this phenomenon an involuntary rest pause which he emphasized
was due to neural fatigue and not muscular fatigue. During this
brief pause, perhaps a half second in duration, inhibition dissipates. Performance is then allowed to continue until inhibition
builds up again and another rest pause occurs.

Eysenck (1973b) proposed that "human beings differ with respect to the speed with which reactive inhibition is produced, the
strength of reactive inhibition and the speed with which reactive
inhibition is dissipated" (p. 126). In relating this statement to
introversion, extroversion, and neuroticism, Eysenck (1973b)
elaborated:

Individuals in whom reactive inhibition is generated quickly,
in whom strong reactive inhibitions are generated and in
whom reactive inhibition is dissipated slowly are thereby predisposed to develop extraverted patterns of behaviour and to
develop hysterical disorders in cases of neurotic breakdown;
conversely, individuals in whom reactive inhibition is generated slowly, in whom weak reactive inhibitions are generated
and in whom reactive inhibition is dissipated quickly, are
thereby predisposed to develop introverted patterns of behaviour and to develop dysthymic disorders in cases of neurotic breakdown (p. 126).

INTROVERSION-EXTROVERSION AND CONDITIONABILITY

Eysenck (1973a) predicted, on the basis of inhibitory-excitatory characteristics, that introverts would condition more readily than extroverts. Despite the failure of some researchers to find a positive correlation between introversion and ease of conditioning, Eysenck cautioned that this does not weaken his prediction. The positive correlation can only be obtained if certain conditioning parameters are employed. Eysenck proposed that conditioning in introverts is favored with partial reinforcement, a weak UCS, and a short CS-UCS interval. First, inhibition is produced during the CS-only trials in partial reinforcement procedures. Introverts are favored under this condition because they develop only a small amount of inhibition, which dissipates quickly. The extrovert, on the other hand, develops a large amount of inhibition, which dissipates slowly. Second, introverts condition better than extroverts when a weak UCS is used because they have lower sensory thresholds. Conditioned responses to low levels of stimulation should be stronger for the introvert than for the extrovert. Eysenck also asserted that responses to a weak UCS habituate quickly and produce inhibition. This inhibition should be weaker in introverts than in extroverts. Third, Eysenck argued that a short CS-UCS interval facilitates conditioning in introverts because their more sensitive nervous system can respond to a rapid rate of presentation. In addition, reactive inhibition would accumulate in the extrovert's nervous system when a short CS-UCS interval is used because of the slow rate at which the extrovert dissipates inhibition.

A study by Levey (cited in Eysenck, 1967, p. 121) was designed to determine the effects of reinforcement schedule, UCS intensity, and CS-UCS interval on the eye-blink conditioning performance of introverts and extroverts. As expected, Levey found that when conditions favorable to introverts were employed; that is, partial reinforcement, a weak UCS, and a short CS-UCS interval, introverts conditioned more readily than extroverts. On the other hand, when continuous reinforcement, a strong UCS, and a long CS-UCS interval were used, extroverts conditioned better than introverts. This experiment stressed the necessity of selecting appropriate conditioning parameters for testing Eysenck's hypothesis. If reinforcement schedule, strength of the UCS, and duration of the CS-UCS interval are randomly selected, the results may not indicate significant differences in conditionability between introverts and extroverts.

Franks (in Eysenck, 1970, p. 92) also tested Eysenck's hypothesis that introverts condition better than extroverts. Franks
used introverted and extroverted neurotics in one study and introverted and extroverted normals for another investigation. The
data for the normal and neurotic subgroups indicated no significant differences in eye-blink conditioning so Franks combined the
data for these two groups. Analysis revealed that the introverts
showed twice as many conditioned responses as the extroverts.
These results supported Eysenck's predictions.

EYSENCK'S BIOLOGICAL THEORY OF PERSONALITY

In 1967, Eysenck proposed that differences in the equilibrium
between excitation and inhibition in introverts and extroverts
were related to differences in the degree of excitation of the ascending reticular activating system (ARAS) of the brain. He also
related the normality-neuroticism variable of his personality theory
to a conglomerate of brain structures called the visceral brain
(VB), which is regarded as the mediator of emotional reactivity.
The interaction between these brain structures is illustrated in
Figure 32. The ARAS is responsible for the efficiency of the cortex in learning, wakefulness, conditioning, attention, and concen-
tration. The ascending afferent pathways transmit information
from the body's sensory receptors to the brain. The reticular
formation provides an alternative pathway for the conduction of
impulses to the cortex (Gooch, 1963). These impulses enter the
reticular formation via collaterals from the ascending afferent pathways and are projected over a wide area of the cortex (Figure 33).
It is the activity of the ARAS, therefore, that determines the degree of cortical excitation. Another portion of the reticular formation, called the 'recruiting system,' exerts an active inhibitory
influence on behavior. Eysenck (1967) postulated "a higher level
of arousal in introverts and a higher level of inhibition in extra-
verts" (p. 241). Hence, the reticular formation provides a phy-
siological-structural basis for the concepts of inhibition and excitation and in turn, for the variables of introversion and extraversion.
The visceral brain structures exert their effect through the
autonomic nervous system, for example, through the glandular,
respiratory, circulatory, and digestive systems. Eysenck proposed that individuals who have high emotional reactivity; that is,
who have a low threshold of visceral brain activation, are susceptible to neuroticism. A low level of visceral brain activation (high

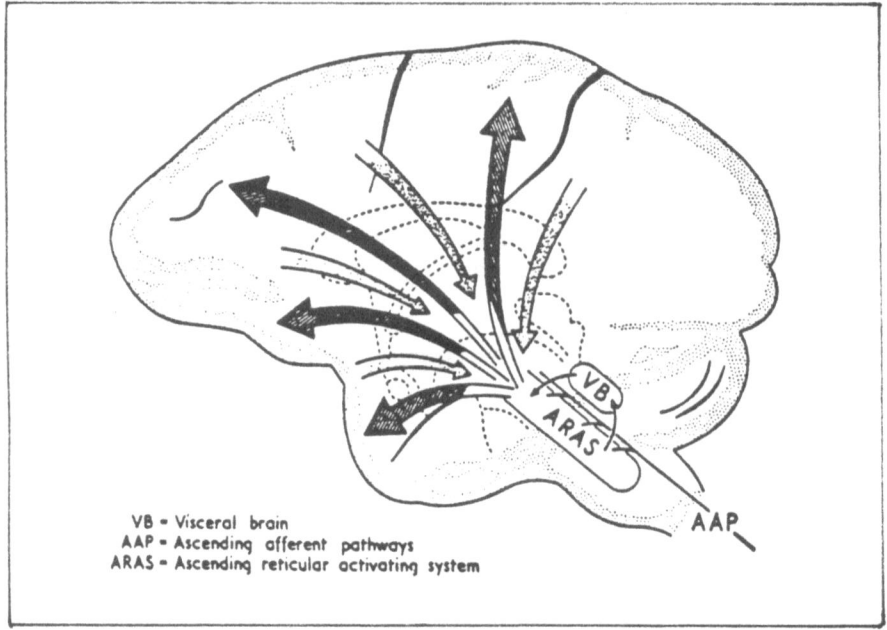

VB = Visceral brain
AAP = Ascending afferent pathways
ARAS = Ascending reticular activating system

AAP

Figure 32. Diagrammatic representation of mutual interaction of reticular formation, visceral brain, and cortex. Direct arousing effects of V.B. stimulation are not indicated in this figure. From *The biological basis of personality*, by H. J. Eysenck. Springfield, Il.: Charles C. Thomas, 1967, p. 231.

threshold) is characteristic of normals. Table 4 illustrates the relation of ARAS arousal and VB activation to intraverted, extraverted, neurotic, and normal personality types.

SOKOLOV'S THEORY OF ATTENTION

Sokolov (in Eysenck, 1967, pp. 249-250) has proposed a model to explain the phenomenon of attention — cortical arousal. According to this model, a neuronal screening system in the cortex stores information such as intensity, duration, and order of presentation of stimuli. The screening system analyzes all incoming stimuli by comparing them to the neuronal traces of previously received stimuli. If a neuronal match does not exist in the cortex

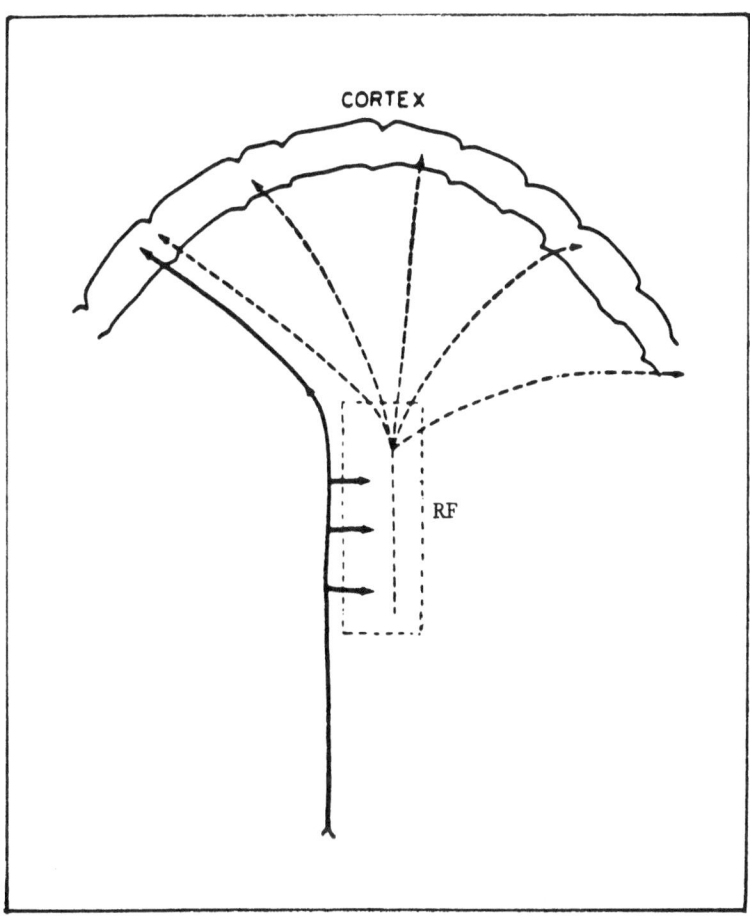

Figure 33. This diagram illustrates the function of the reticular
formation (R.F.) as an alternative pathway for impulses proceed-
ing from the periphery to the cortex. From "The Influence of
Stimulant and Depressant Drugs on the Central Nervous System,"
by R. N. Gooch. In H. J. Eysenck (ed.), *Experiments with
drugs: Studies in the relation between personality, learning
theory and drug action.* New York: Macmillan, 1963, p. 360.

for a particular stimulus, the reticular activating system is stimulated by impulses from the cortex. In turn, the reticular formation arouses the cortex and evokes an orienting reaction. Novel
stimuli or stimuli that are significant to an organism will initiate

TABLE 4. Biological Basis of Personality

Dimensional position	Level of ARAS arousal	Level of VB activation
Normal introvert	High	Low
Normal extrovert	Low	Low
Neurotic introvert (Dysthymic)	High	High
Neurotic extrovert (Hysteric)	Low[a]	High

From *Beneath the Mask: An Introduction to Theories of Personality*, by C. F. Monte. New York: Praeger, 1977, p. 627.
[a]Note that the *neurotic* extravert's ARAS arousal is higher than the normal extrovert's ARAS arousal because of the breakdown of separation between ARAS and VB functioning in states of high (neurotic) emotion. But the extrovert's characteristic ARAS arousal level is always lower than the introvert's level, and is therefore simply listed as "low." Based on Eysenck (1967).

this excitatory mechanism in the cortex. In the case of familiar stimuli, a match is found in the existing neuronal traces in the cortex and inhibitory impulses are sent to the reticular formation. Arousal is inhibited and an orienting reaction is not evoked. Pavlov observed that "the weak nervous system [introvert] is particularly liable to display persisting orienting reflexes" (in Eysenck, 1967, pp. 251-252). Orienting reactions are usually indicated by changes in physiological responses such as heart rate, respiration rate, and galvanic skin responses (Das, 1978, p. 34).

DIFFERENTIAL EFFECTS OF STIMULANT AND DEPRESSANT DRUGS ON INTROVERTS AND EXTROVERTS

Extending on the ARAS theory of intraversion-extroversion, it is predictable that:

Stimulant drugs lead to greater arousal and hence to more introverted behaviour, while depressant drugs lead to greater inhibition and hence to more extraverted behaviour . . . . Introverts, being in a comparatively high state of cortical arousal, would require less of a stimulant drug than extroverts to reach a specified state of excitation, but would require more of a depressant drug to reach a specified state of inhibition. In other words, introverts have higher sedation thresholds than extroverts, but extroverts have higher excitation thresholds (Eysenck, 1967, p. 265).

A sedation threshold measure may be obtained by determining the amount of a drug that must be injected into an individual, at a known rate, to produce specific EEG changes and slurred speech. This particular method was used by Shagass and Kerenyi (cited in Eysenck, 1967). These researchers found that introverts required less of a depressant drug than extroverts which supported Eysenck's prediction of a positive correlation between sedation threshold and introversion. Shagass and Kerenyi also demonstrated that hysterics (extroverted neurotics) had lower sedation thresholds than dysthymics (introverted neurotics) which further supports Eysenck's hypothesis.

YERKES-DODSON LAW

While the high cortical arousal of the introvert is said to result in better conditioning performance, the Yerkes-Dodson law (in Eysenck, 1967, 1970) seems to take exception to this notion. It states that performance is poor at both low and high levels of drive or arousal because the organism is either undermotivated or so highly aroused that its behavior is disorganized and fragmented. Optimum performance is achieved at intermediate levels of drive. This law is depicted in Figure 34.

The effect of different stimulus intensities on performance can be predicted from and accounted for on the basis of the Yerkes-Dodson law. Eysenck (1957) stated:

When a very weak electric shock was used as a drive, the animal would learn only slowly. When a very strong shock was used, the very strength of the stimulus appeared to interfere with the learning and performance of the animal. Intermediate degrees of shock were found to produce the best results (p. 95).

The observation that performance improves as arousal increases, up to a certain point, bears some relation to Teplov's strong-weak

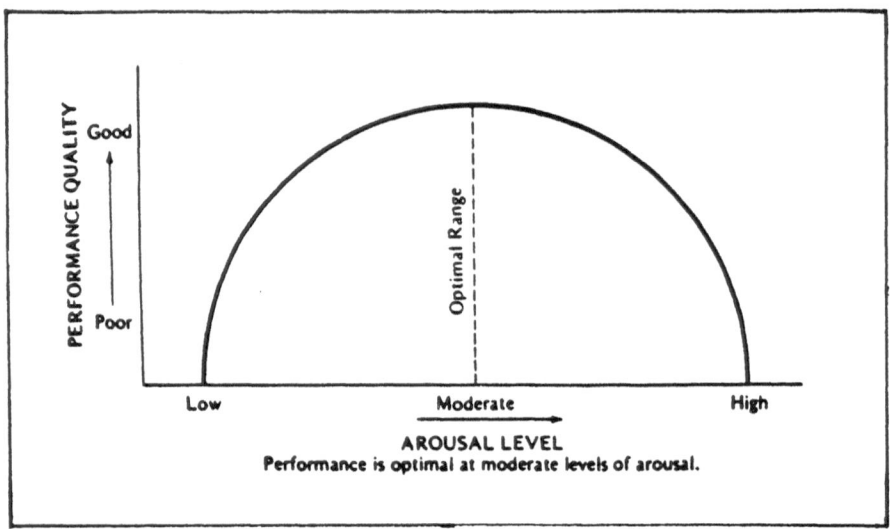

Figure 34. Inverted-U law of motivation and performance. From
Beneath the mask: An introduction to theories of personality, by
C. F. Monte. New York: Praeger, 1977, p. 628.

nervous system concept and to Pavlov's concept of transmarginal
inhibition. It appears that the previously discussed results of
Levey's investigation in which the variables of reinforcement schedule, UCS intensity, and CS-UCS interval were manipulated can
be explained more easily by the Yerkes-Dodson law than by the
inhibition-excitation model. Monte (1977) stated that the law is
especially applicable to Levey's finding that extroverts conditioned
better with a strong UCS and that introverts conditioned better
when the UCS was weak:

> If UCS intensity is conceptualized as a form of arousal, the
> Yerkes-Dodson law predicts that introverts, having a higher
> level of initial arousal, will perform poorly with the additional
> arousal provided by a strong UCS. Extr[o]verts, on the
> other hand, profit from the arousal increment because their
> initial cortical arousal is low (p. 630).

References

Achenbach, T. M. *Developmental psychopathology*. New York: Ronald Press, 1974.

Adams, J. A. *Learning and memory: An introduction*. Homewood, IL: Dorsey Press, 1976.

Apsche, J., Bacevich, R., Axelrod, S., and Keach, S. *Use of an eyescreen (blindfold) as a timeout procedure*. Paper presented at the Eleventh Annual Gatlinburg Conference on Mental Retardation, Gatlinburg, Tennessee, March, 1978.

Averill, J. R., and Rosenn, M. Vigilant and nonvigilant coping strategies and psychophysiological stress reactions during the anticipation of electric shock. *Journal of Personality and Social Psychology*, 1972, *23*, 128-141.

Azrin, N. H. Effects of punishment intensity during variable-interval reinforcement. *Journal of the Experimental Analysis of Behavior*, 1960, *3*, 123-142.

Badia, P., and Culbertson, S. Behavioral effects of signalled vs. unsignalled shock during escape training in the rat. *Journal of Comparative and Physiological Psychology*, 1970, *72*, 216-222.

Badia, P., Suter, S., and Lewis, P. Preference for warned shock: Information and/or preparation. *Psychological Reports*, 1967, *20*, 271-274.

Bandura, A. *Principles of behavior modification*. New York: Holt, Rinehart and Winston, 1969.

Barlow, D. H., Leitenberg, H., and Agras, W. S. The experimental control of sexual deviation through manipulation of the noxious scene in covert sensitization. *Journal of Abnormal Psychology*, 1969, *74*, 596-601.

Barmann, B. C., and Murray, W. J. Suppression of inappropriate sexual behavior by facial screening. *Behavior Therapy*, 1981, *12*, 730-735.

Barmann, B. C., and Vitali, D. L. Facial screening to eliminate trichotillomania in developmentally disabled persons. *Behavior Therapy*, 1982, *13*, 735-742.

Benedict, J. O., and Ayres, J. J. B. Factors affecting conditioning in a truly random control procedure in the rat. *Journal of Comparative and Physiological Psychology*, 1972, *78*, 323-330.

Berecz, J. Modification of smoking behavior through self-administered punishment of imagined behavior: A new approach to aversion therapy. *Journal of Consulting and Clinical Psychology*, 1972, *38*, 244-250.

Berlyne, D. E. *Conflict, arousal and curiosity*. New York: McGraw-Hill, 1960.

Bersh, P. J. Eysenck's theory of incubation: A critical analysis. *Behaviour Research and Therapy*, 1980, *18*, 11-17.

Black, A. H., Osborne, B., and Ristow, W. C. A note on the operant conditioning of autonomic responses. In H. Davis and H. M. B. Hurwitz (eds.), *Operant-Pavlovian interactions*. Hillsdale, NJ: Lawrence Erlbaum, 1977.

Blakiston's Gould medical dictionary (3d ed.). New York: McGraw-Hill, 1972.

Bolles, R. C. Species-specific defense reactions and avoidance learning. *Psychological Review*, 1970, 77, 32-48.

Bolles, R. C., and McGillis, D. B. The non-operant nature of the bar-press escape response. *Psychonomic Science*, 1968, *11*, 261-262.

Bolles, R. C., and Warren, J. A., Jr. Effects of delay on the punishing and reinforcing effects of noise onset and termination. *Journal of Comparative and Physiological Psychology*, 1966, *61*, 475-477.

Bowers, K. S. The effects of UCS temporal uncertainty on heart rate and pain. *Psychophysiology*, 1971, *8*, 382-389.

Brady, J. P., and Esty, J. F. Social parameters of anxiety in the rat. *Recent Advances in Biological Psychiatry*, 1963, *5*, 175-183.

Breland, K., and Breland, M. The misbehavior of organisms. *American Psychologist*, 1961, *16*, 681-684.

Brown, J. S., and Jacobs, A. The role of fear in the motivation and acquisition of responses. *Journal of Experimental Psychology*, 1949, *39*, 747-759.

Brown, P., and Jenkins, H. M. Autoshaping of the pigeon's keypeck. *Journal of the Experimental Analysis of Behavior*, 1968, *11*, 1-8.

Bugelski, B. R. *The psychology of learning applied to teaching*, (2d ed.). Indianapolis: Bobbs-Merrill, 1971.

Butterfield, W. H. Electric shock — Safety factors when used for the aversive conditioning of humans. *Behavior Therapy*, 1975, *6*, 98-110.

Carlin, A. S., and Armstrong, H. E., Jr. Aversive conditioning: Learning or dissonance reduction? *Journal of Consulting and Clinical Psychology*, 1968, *32*, 674-678.

Church, R. M. The role of fear in punishment. In J. R. Braun (chm.), *The effects of punishment on behavior*. Symposium presented at the meeting of the American Psychological Association, New York, September, 1966.

Clark, J. W., and Bindra, D. Individual differences in pain threshold. *Canadian Journal of Psychology*, 1956, *10*, 69-76.

Craighead, W. E., Kazdin, A. E., and Mahoney, M. J. *Behavior modification: Principles, issues, and applications* (2d ed.). Boston: Houghton Mifflin, 1981.

Das, J. P. Attention. In J. P. Das and D. Baine (eds.), *Mental retardation for special educators*. Springfield, IL: Charles C. Thomas, 1978.

Davis, H. Response characteristics and control during leverpress escape. In H. Davis and H. M. B. Hurwitz (eds.), *Operant-Pavlovian interactions*. Hillsdale, NJ: Lawrence Erlbaum, 1977.

Davis, H., and Burton, J. The measurement of response force during a leverpress shock escape procedure in rats. *Journal of the Experimental Analysis of Behavior*, 1974, *22*, 433-440.

Davis, H., Hirschorn, P., and Hurwitz, H. M. B. Lever holding behavior during a leverlift shock escape procedure. *Animal Learning and Behavior*, 1973, *1*, 215-218.

Davis, H., and Kenney, S. Some effects of different test cages on response "strategies" during leverpress escape. *Psychological Record*, 1975, *25*, 535-543.

Davis, H., Porter, J. W., Burton, J., and Levine, S. Sex and strain differences in leverpress shock escape behavior. *Physiological Psychology*, 1976, *4*, 351-356.

Deitz, S. M., and Hummel, J. H. *Discipline in the schools*. Englewood Cliffs, NJ: Educational Technology Publications, 1978.

Demetral, G. D., and Lutzker, J. R. The parameters of facial screening in treating self-injurious behavior. *Behavior Research of Severe Developmental Disabilities*, 1980, *1*, 261-277.

Derevensky, J. L. Children's fears: A developmental comparison of normal and exceptional children. *Journal of Genetic Psychology*, 1979, *135*, 11-21.

Devany, J., and Rincover, A. Self-stimulatory behavior and sensory reinforcement. In R. L. Koegel, A. Rincover, and A. L. Egel (eds.), *Educating and understanding autistic children*. San Diego: College-Hill, 1982.

Dunham, P. J. *Experimental psychology: Theory and practice*. New York: Harper and Row, 1977.

Ellis, H. C. *Fundamentals of human learning, memory, and cognition* (2d ed.). Dubuque, IA: Wm. C. Brown, 1978.

Eysenck, H. J. *The dynamics of anxiety and hysteria: An experimental application of modern learning theory to psychiatry*. London: Routledge and Kegan Paul, 1957.

Eysenck, H. J. *The biological basis of personality*. Springfield, IL: Charles C. Thomas, 1967.

Eysenck, H. J. A theory of the incubation of anxiety/fear responses. *Behaviour Research and Therapy*, 1968, *6*, 309-321.

Eysenck, H. J. *Crime and personality*. London: Paladin, 1970.

Eysenck, H. J. Conditioning, introversion-extraversion and the strength of the nervous system. In H. J. Eysenck (ed.), *Eysenck on extraversion*. London: Crosby Lockwood Staples, 1973 (a).

Eysenck, H. J. Cortical inhibition, figural aftereffect and theory of personality. In H. J. Eysenck (ed.), *Eysenck on extraversion*. London: Crosby Lockwood Staples, 1973 (b).

Eysenck, H. J. The learning theory model of neurosis — a new approach. *Behaviour Research and Therapy*, 1976, *14*, 251-267.

Eysenck, H. J. The conditioning model of neurosis. *The Behavioral and Brain Sciences*, 1979, *2*, 155-199.

Feldman, M. P., and MacCulloch, M. J. The application of anticipatory avoidance learning to the treatment of homosexuality. *Behavior Research and Therapy*, 1965, *2*, 165-183.

Friedman, S. F., and Ader, R. A. Parameters relevant to the experimental production of stress in the mouse. *Psychosomatic Medicine*, 1965, *27*, 27-30.

Galbraith, D. A., Byrick, R. J., and Rutledge, J. T. An aversive conditioning approach to the inhibition of chronic vomiting. *Canadian Psychiatric Association Journal*, 1970, *15*, 311-313.

Garcia, J., Kimeldorf, D. J., and Koelling, R. A. Conditioned aversion to saccharin from exposure to gamma radiation. *Science*, 1955, *122*, 157-158.

Garcia, J., and Koelling, R. A. Relation of cue to consequence in avoidance learning. In M. E. P. Seligman and J. L. Hager (eds.), Biological boundaries of learning. New York: Appleton-Century-Crofts, 1972.

Garcia, J., McGowan, B. K., and Green, K. F. Biological constraints on conditioning. In A. H. Black and W. F. Prokasy (eds.), Classical conditioning II: Current research and theory. New York: Appleton-Century-Crofts, 1972.

Geer, J. H. A test of the classical conditioning model of emotion: The use of non-painful aversive stimuli as UCSs in a conditioning procedure. Journal of Personality and Social Psychology, 1968, 10, 148-156.

Gelfand, D. M., and Hartmann, D. P. Child behavior analysis and therapy. New York: Pergamon, 1975.

Gelfand, S. The relationship of birth order to pain tolerance. Journal of Clinical Psychology, 1963, 19, 406.

Gelfand, S. The relation of experimental pain tolerance to pain threshold. Canadian Journal of Psychology, 1964, 18, 36-42.

Gelfand, S., Ullmann, L. P., and Krasner, L. The placebo response: An experimental approach. Journal of Nervous and Mental Disease, 1963, 136, 379-387.

Glass, D. C., and Singer, J. E. Urban condition: Experiments on noise and social stressor. New York: Academic Press, 1972.

Glynn, C. J., and Lloyd, J. W. The diurnal variation in perception of pain. Proceedings of the Royal Society of Medicine, 1976, 69, 369-372.

Gooch, R. N. The influence of stimulant and depressant drugs on the central nervous system. In H. J. Eysenck (ed.), Experiments with drugs: Studies in the relation between personality, learning theory and drug action. New York: Macmillan, 1963.

Grant, D. A., and Schipper, L. M. The acquisition and extinction of conditioned eyelid responses as a function of the percentage of fixed-ratio random reinforcement. Journal of Experimental Psychology, 1952, 43, 313-320.

Gray, J. A. Strength of the nervous system as a dimension of personality in man: A review of work from the laboratory of B. M. Teplov. In J. A. Gray (ed.), Pavlov's typology. Oxford: Pergamon, 1964.

Gray, J. A. Strength of the nervous system, introversion-extroversion, conditionability and arousal. Behaviour Research and Therapy, 1967, 5, 151-169.

Hall, J. F. *Classical conditioning and instrumental learning: A contemporary approach.* Philadelphia: Lippincott, 1976.

Hallam, R., and Rachman, S. Theoretical problems of aversion therapy. *Behaviour Research and Therapy*, 1972, *10*, 341-353.

Hallam, R. S., and Rachman, S. Current status of aversion therapy. In M. Hersen, R. M. Eisler, and P. M. Miller (eds.), *Progress in behavior modification* (Vol. 2). New York: Academic Press, 1976.

Hallam, R., Rachman, S., and Falkowski, W. Subjective, attitudinal and physiological effects of electrical aversion therapy. *Behaviour Research and Therapy*, 1972, *10*, 1-13.

Hergenhahn, B. R. *An introduction to theories of learning.* Englewood Cliffs, NJ: Prentice-Hall, 1976.

Hilgard, E. R., and Marquis, D. G. *Conditioning and learning.* New York: Appleton-Century-Crofts, 1940.

Holland, P. C., and Rescorla, R. A. The effect of two ways of devaluing the unconditioned stimulus after first- and second-order appetitive conditioning. *Journal of Experimental Psychology: Animal Behavior Processes*, 1975, *1*, 355-363 (a).

Holland, P. C., and Rescorla, R. A. Second-order conditioning with food unconditioned stimulus. *Journal of Comparative and Physiological Psychology*, 1975, *88*, 459-467 (b).

Hurwitz, H. M. B., and Roberts, A. E. Aversively controlled behavior and the analysis of conditioned suppression. In H. Davis and H. M. B. Hurwitz (eds.), *Operant-Pavlovian interactions*. Hillsdale, NJ: Lawrence Erlbaum, 1977.

Johnston, J. M. Punishment of human behavior. *American Psychologist*, 1972, *27*, 1033-1054.

Kalat, J. W., and Rozin, P. Role of interference in taste aversion learning. *Journal of Comparative and Physiological Psychology*, 1971, *77*, 53-58.

Kalish, H. I. Strength of fear as a function of the number of acquisition and extinction trials. *Journal of Experimental Psychology*, 1954, *47*, 1-9.

Kamin, L. J. The effects of termination of the CS and avoidance of the US on avoidance learning. *Journal of Comparative and Physiological Psychology*, 1956, *49*, 420-424.

Kanfer, F. H., and Phillips, J. S. *Learning foundations of behavior therapy.* New York: Wiley, 1970.

Kazdin, A. E. *Behavior modification in applied settings* (rev. ed.). Homewood, IL: Dorsey Press, 1980.

Kimmel, E., and Kimmel, H. D. A replication of operant conditioning of the GSR. *Journal of Experimental Psychology*, 1963, *65*, 212-213.

Kremer, E. F. Random and traditional control procedures in CER conditioning in the rat. *Journal of Comparative and Physiological Psychology*, 1971, *76*, 441-448.

Kremer, E. F., and Kamin, L. J. The truly random control procedure: Associative or nonassociative effects in rats. *Journal of Comparative and Physiological Psychology*, 1971, *74*, 203-210.

Kushner, M. Faradic aversive controls in clinical practice. In C. Neuringer and J. L. Michael (eds.), *Behavior modification in clinical psychology*. New York: Appleton-Century-Crofts, 1970.

Lang, P. J., and Melamed, B. G. Avoidance conditioning therapy of an infant with chronic ruminative vomiting. *Journal of Abnormal Psychology*, 1969, *74*, 1-8.

Laverty, S. G. Aversion therapies in the treatment of alcoholism. *Psychosomatic Medicine*, 1966, *23*, 651-666.

Leitenberg, H. Is time-out from positive reinforcement an aversive event? *Psychological Bulletin*, 1965, *64*, 428-441 (a).

Leitenberg, H. Response initiation and response termination: Analysis of effects of punishment and escape contingencies. *Psychological Reports*, 1965, *16*, 569-575 (b).

Logan, D. L., and Turnage, J. R. Ethical considerations in the use of faradic aversion therapy. *Behavioral Engineering*, 1975, *3*, 29-34.

Lovibond, S. H. Intermittent reinforcement in behaviour therapy. *Behaviour Research and Therapy*, 1963, *1*, 127-132.

Lovibond, S. H. Aversive control of behavior. *Behavior Therapy*, 1970, *1*, 80-91.

Lutzker, J. R. Reducing self-injurious behavior by facial screening. *American Journal of Mental Deficiency*, 1978, *82*, 510-513.

Lutzker, J. R., and Spencer, T. *Punishment of self-injurious behavior in retardates by brief application of a harmless face cover.* Paper presented at the meeting of the American Psychological Association, New Orleans, September, 1974.

Lutzker, J. R., and Wesch, D. Facial screening: History and critical review. *Australia and New Zealand Journal of Developmental Disabilities*, in press.

Lynn, R., and Eysenck, H. J. Tolerance for pain, extraversion and neuroticism. *Perceptual and Motor Skills*, 1961, *12*, 161-162.

Mackintosh, N. J. Stimulus selection: Learning to ignore stimuli that predict no change in reinforcement. In R. A. Hindle and J. S. Hindle (eds.), *Constraints on learning*. London: Academic Press, 1973.

Manning, A. A., Schneiderman, N., and Lordahl, D. S. Delay versus trace heart-rate classical discrimination conditioning in rabbits as a function of interstimulus interval. *Journal of Experimental Psychology*, 1969, *80*, 225-230.

Marks, I., Gelder, M., and Bancroft, J. Sexual deviants two years after electrical aversion. *British Journal of Psychiatry*, 1970, *117*, 173-185.

McConaghy, N. Aversive therapy of homosexuality: Measures of efficacy. *American Journal of Psychiatry*, 1971, *127*, 1221-1224.

McConaghy, N. Aversion therapy. *Seminars in Psychiatry*, 1972, *4*, 139-144.

McGonigle, J. J., Duncan, D., Cordisco, L., and Barrett, R. P. Visual screening: An alternative method for reducing stereotypic behaviors. *Journal of Applied Behavior Analysis*, 1982, *15*, 461-467.

Mikulas, W. L. *Behavior modification*. New York: Harper and Row, 1978.

Miller, N. E. Learnable drives and rewards. In S. S. Stevens (ed.), *Handbook of experimental psychology*. New York: Wiley, 1951.

Miller, N. E., and Carmona, A. Modification of a visceral response, salivation in thirsty dogs, by instrumental training with water reward. *Journal of Comparative and Physiological Psychology*, 1967, *63*, 1-6.

Miller, N. E., and DiCara, L. Instrumental learning of heart rate changes in curarized rats: Shaping and specificity to discriminative stimuli. *Journal of Comparative and Physiological Psychology*, 1967, *63*, 12-19.

Monte, C. F. *Beneath the mask: An introduction to theories of personality*. New York: Praeger, 1977.

Moss, G. R., Rada, R. T., and Appel, J. B. Positive control as an alternative to aversion therapy. *Journal of Behavior Therapy and Experimental Psychiatry*, 1970, *1*, 291-294.

Mowrer, O. H. On the dual nature of learning — A re-interpretation of 'conditioning' and 'problem solving'. *Harvard Educational Review*, 1947, *17*, 102-148.

O'Leary, K. D., and Wilson, G. T. *Behavior therapy: Application and outcome*. Englewood Cliffs, NJ: Prentice-Hall, 1975.

Pavlov, I. P. *Conditioned reflexes: An investigation into the physiological activity of the cortex*. New York: Dover, 1927.

Pavlov, I. P. *Lectures on conditioned reflexes*. New York: International Publishers, 1928.

Perkins, C. C. The stimulus conditions which follow learned responses. *Psychological Review*, 1955, *62*, 341-348.

Pervin, L. A. The need to predict and control under conditions of threat. *Journal of Personality*, 1963, *31*, 570-587.

Quattlebaum, L. F. "A theory of the incubation of anxiety/fear responses": An alternative. *Psychological Reports*, 1970, *26*, 747-749.

Quinsey, V. L. Conditioned suppression with no CS-US contingency in the rat. *Canadian Journal of Psychology*, 1971, *25*, 69-82.

Rachlin, H. *Introduction to modern behaviorism* (2d ed.). San Francisco: Freeman, 1970.

Rachman, S., and Teasdale, J. D. Aversion therapy: An appraisal. In C. M. Franks (ed.), *Behavior therapy: Appraisal and status*. New York: McGraw-Hill, 1969.

Reese, H. W., and Lipsitt, L. P. *Experimental child psychology*. New York: Academic Press, 1970.

Rescorla, R. A. Pavlovian conditioning and its proper control procedures. *Psychological Review*, 1967, *74*, 71-80.

Rescorla, R. A. Probability of shock in the presence and absence of the CS in fear conditioning. *Journal of Comparative and Physiological Psychology*, 1968, *66*, 1-5.

Rescorla, R. A. Conditioned inhibition of fear resulting from negative CS-US contingencies. *Journal of Comparative and Physiological Psychology*, 1969, *67*, 504-509.

Rescorla, R. A. Pavlovian second-order conditioning: Some implications for instrumental behavior. In H. Davis and H. M. B. Hurwitz (eds.), *Operant-Pavlovian interactions*. Hillsdale, NJ: Lawrence Erlbaum, 1977.

Rescorla, R. A., and Solomon, R. L. Two-process learning theory: Relationships between Pavlovian conditioning and instrumental learning. *Psychological Review*, 1967, *74*, 151-182.

Revusky, S. The role of interference in association over a delay. In W. K. Honig and P. H. R. James (eds.), *Animal memory*. New York: Academic Press, 1971.

Rimm, D. C., and Masters, J. C. *Behavior therapy: Techniques and empirical findings*. New York: Academic Press, 1974.

Rincover, A. Sensory extinction: A procedure for eliminating self-stimulatory behavior in developmentally disabled children. *Journal of Abnormal Child Psychology*, 1978, *6*, 299-310.

Rincover, A., Cook, R., Peoples, A., and Packard, D. Sensory extinction and sensory reinforcement principles for programming multiple adaptive behavior change. *Journal of Applied Behavior Analysis*, 1979, *12*, 221-233.

Rincover, A., and Devany, J. M. *Experimental analysis of ethical issues: I. Using self-stimulation as a reinforcer in the treatment of developmentally delayed children.* Paper presented at the 12th Annual Meeting, Association for the Advancement of Behavior Therapy, Chicago, 1978.

Rincover, A., and Devany, J. M. *The nature and role of side effects in research on ethics.* Paper presented at the Association for Behavior Analysis Annual Meeting, Dearborn, Michigan, 1979.

Rincover, A., and Koegel, R. L. Research on the education of autistic children: Recent advances and future directions. In B. B. Lahey and A. E. Kazdin (eds.), *Advances in clinical child psychology* (Vol. 1). New York: Plenum Press, 1977.

Rincover, A., Newsom, C. D., Lovaas, O. I., and Koegel, R. L. Some motivational properties of sensory stimulation in psychotic children. *Journal of Experimental Child Psychology*, 1977, *24*, 312-323.

Rogers, E. J., and Vilkin, B. Diurnal variation in sensory and pain thresholds correlated with mood states. *Journal of Clinical Psychiatry*, 1978, *39*, 431-432; 438.

Scholander, T. Treatment of an unusual case of compulsive behavior by aversive stimulation. *Behavior Therapy*, 1972, *3*, 290-293.

Schwartz, B. *Psychology of learning and behavior.* New York: W. W. Norton, 1978.

Schwitzgebel, R. K., and Traugott, M. Initial note on the placebo effect of machines. *Behavioral Science*, 1968, *13*, 267-273.

Seligman, M. E. P. Chronic fear produced by unpredictable electric shock. *Journal of Comparative and Physiological Psychology*, 1968, *66*, 402-411.

Seligman, M. E. P. *Helplessness: On depression, development, and death.* San Francisco: Freeman, 1975.

Seligman, M. E. P., and Binik, Y. M. The safety signal hypothesis. In H. Davis and H. M. B. Hurwitz (eds.), *Operant-Pavlovian interactions.* Hillsdale, NJ: Lawrence Erlbaum, 1977.

Seligman, M. E. P., and Hager, J. L. (eds.). *Biological boundaries of learning.* New York: Appleton-Century-Crofts, 1972.

Seligman, M. E. P., and Johnston, J. C. A cognitive theory of avoidance learning. In F. J. McGuigan and D. B. Lumsden (eds.), *Contemporary approaches to conditioning and learning.* New York: Wiley, 1973.

Seligman, M. E. P., and Meyer, B. Chronic fear produced by unpredictable shock. *Journal of Comparative and Physiological Psychology*, 1970, *73*, 202-207.

Shearn, D. Operant conditioning of the heart rate response. *Science*, 1962, *137*, 530-531.

Singh, N. N. The effects of facial screening on infant self-injury. *Journal of Behavior Therapy and Experimental Psychiatry*, 1980, *11*, 131-134.

Singh, N. N., Beale, I. L., and Dawson, M. J. Duration of facial screening and suppression of self-injurious behaviour: Analysis using an alternating treatments design. *Behavioral Assessment*, 1981, *3*, 411-420.

Singh, N. N., Winton, A. S., and Dawson, M. J. Suppression of antisocial behavior by facial screening using multiple baseline and alternating treatments designs. *Behavior Therapy*, 1982, *13*, 511-520.

Staats, A. W. (ed.). *Human learning: Studies extending conditioning principles to complex behavior*. New York: Holt, Rinehart and Winston, 1964.

Staats, A. W., and Staats, C. K. *Complex human behavior: A systematic extension of learning principles*. New York: Holt, Rinehart and Winston, 1963.

Stumphauzer, J. S. A low-cost "bug-in-the-ear" sound system for modification of therapist, parent, and patient behavior. *Behavior Therapy*, 1971, *2*, 249-250.

Trowill, J. A. Instrumental conditioning of the heart rate in the curarized rat. *Journal of Comparative and Physiological Psychology*, 1967, *63*, 7-11.

Vogler, R. E., Lunde, S. E., Johnson, G. R., and Martin, P. L. Electrical aversion conditioning with chronic alcoholics. *Journal of Consulting and Clinical Psychology*, 1970, *34*, 302-307.

von Holst, E., and von Saint Paul, U. On the functional organisation of drives. *Animal Behaviour*, 1963, *11*, 1-20.

Wahlsten, D. L., and Cole, M. Classical and avoidance training of leg flexion in the dog. In A. H. Black and W. F. Prokasy (eds.), *Classical conditioning II: Current research and theory*. New York: Appleton-Century-Crofts, 1972.

Walters, G. C., and Grusec, J. E. *Punishment*. San Francisco: Freeman, 1977.

Watson, J. B., and Rayner, R. Conditioned emotional reactions. *Journal of Experimental Psychology*, 1920, *3*, 1-14.

Watson, J. B., and Rayner, R. Conditioned emotional reactions. In A. W. Staats (ed.), *Human learning: Studies extending conditioning principles to complex behavior*. New York: Holt, Rinehart and Winston, 1964.

Weisman, R. G. On the role of the reinforcer in associative learning. In H. Davis and H. M. B. Hurwitz, (eds.), *Operant-Pavlovian interactions*. Hillsdale, NJ: Lawrence Erlbaum, 1977.

Weiss, J. M. Somatic effects of predictable and unpredictable shock. *Psychosomatic Medicine*, 1970, *32*, 397-408.

Weiss, J. M. Effects of coping behavior with and without a feedback signal on stress pathology in rats. *Journal of Comparative and Physiological Psychology*, 1971, *77*, 22-30.

White, G. D. , Nielsen, G. , and Johnson, S. M. Timeout duration and the suppression of deviant behavior in children. *Journal of Applied Behavior Analysis*, 1972, *5*, 111-120.

Wilcoxon, H. C. , Dragoin, W. B. , and Kral, P. A. Illness induced aversions in the rat and quail: Relative salience of visual and gustatory cues. *Science*, 1971, *171*, 826-828.

Williams, J. L. *Operant learning: Procedures for changing behavior*. Monterey, CA: Brooks/Cole, 1973.

Williamson, D. A. , Coon, R. C. , Lemoine, R. L. , and Cohen, C. R. A practical application of sensory extinction for reducing the disruptive classroom behavior of a profoundly retarded child. *School Psychology Review*, 1983, *12*, 205-211.

Wilson, G. T. , and Davison, G. C. Aversion techniques in behavior therapy: Some theoretical and metatheoretical considerations. *Journal of Consulting and Clinical Psychology*, 1969, *33*, 327-329.

Wolpe, J. *Psychotherapy by reciprocal inhibition*. Stanford, CA: Stanford University Press, 1958.

Wolpe, J. *The practice of behavior therapy*. New York: Pergamon, 1969.

Zegiob, L. , Alford, G. S. , and House, A. Response suppressive and generalization effects of facial screening on multiple self-injurious behavior in a retarded boy. *Behavior Therapy*, 1978, *9*, 688.

Zegiob, L. E. , Jenkins, J:, Becker, J. , and Bristow, A. Facial screening: Effects on appropriate and inappropriate behaviors. *Journal of Behavior Therapy and Experimental Psychiatry*, 1976, *7*, 355-357.

Name Index

Achenbach, T. M. 71, 73
Adams, J. A. 2, 95-96
Ader, R. A. 47
Agras, W. S. 93
Alford, G. S. 67, 72
Allport, G. W. 17
Appel, J. B. 36
Apsche, J. 69, 71, 73
Armstrong, H. E., Jr. 86-87
Averill, J. R. 46
Axelrod, S. 69
Ayres, J. J. B. 12
Azrin, N. H. 30

Bacevich, R. 69
Badia, P. 44-46
Bancroft, J. 52, 54, 84
Bandura, A. 36, 55, 88
Barlow, D. H. 93
Barmann, B. C. 66, 68-69, 72, 77
Barrett, R. P. 70
Beale, I. L. 65
Becker, J. 65
Beecher, H. K. 60, 112
Benedict, J. O. 12
Berecz, J. 51
Berlyne, D. E. 44
Bersh, P. J. 90-91
Bindra, D. 59-60
Binik, Y. M. 43-44, 47-48

Black, A. H. 21-22
Bolles, R. C. 34, 38-39, 103
Bonoma, T. V. 87
Bowers, K. S. 47
Brady, J. P. 47
Breland, K. 22
Breland, M. 22
Bristow, A. 65
Brown, J. S. 97
Brown, P. 19
Bucher, B. 49
Bugelski, B. R. 114
Burton, J. 43
Butterfield, W. H. 51, 61-62
Byrick, R. J. 50

Carlin, A. S. 86-87
Carmona, A. 3
Church, R. M. 36
Clark, J. W. 59-60
Cohen, C. R. 76
Cole, M. 95
Cook, R. 69
Coon, R. C. 76
Cordisco, L. 70
Craighead, W. E. 77
Culbertson, S. 46

Das, J. P. 120
Davis, H. 38-43

135

Subject Index

[Safety signal hypothesis]
empirical and logical problems 47-48
empirical support for 46-47
illustrated in the natural
environment 44
in classical conditioning 44
Second-order conditioning
definition 15
minimizing extinction of
first-order conditioning
16
resistance to extinction 15-
16
role in instrumental learning
16-17
standard procedure 15-16
Self-injurious behavior
and sensory extinction 77-
79
effectiveness of facial
screening 65-67
effectiveness of faradic
aversion therapy 49-50
Self-stimulatory behavior
effectiveness of facial
screening 66
effectiveness of sensory extinction 75-80
examples 66, 75-76, 79-80
reinforcing function of 79-
80
Sensory extinction
advantages 77-78
definition 75
description of procedure 75
distinction between extinction and punishment 77
explanation for facial
screening 77
for treating self-injurious
behavior 77-79
for treating self-stimulation
75-80

[Sensory extinction]
limitations 78-79
masking 76
sensory reinforcement 75-80
Sensory inhibition 112
Sokolov's theory of attention
118-120
Species-specific defense reactions (SSDRs). See Bio-
logical theory of escape and
avoidance learning
State theory of aversion therapy 94
Stimulus relevance in conditioning
concurrent interference principle 26-28
evolutionary predisposition
hypothesis 26
examples of 24-25
implications for human research 25
lifetime correlations hypothesis 28
See also Preparedness in classical conditioning
Strong nervous system 110,
112-113

Time-out
and facial screening 69, 73-75
contingent observation 73
duration guidelines 74-75
exclusion time-out 73
respondent and operant ex-
planations 73
seclusion time-out 73
Transmarginal inhibition 112-
113
Two-factor theory explanation
of aversive control of behavior
assumptions 95